Elder Abuse and Neglect

Veronica LoFaso • Lisa Rachmuth
Editors

Elder Abuse and Neglect

A Case-based Guide for Health Care and Elder Justice Professionals

Springer

Editors
Veronica LoFaso (Retired)
Division of Geriatrics and Palliative Medicine
Weill Cornell Medicine
New York, NY, USA

Lisa Rachmuth
Division of Geriatrics and Palliative Medicine
Center for Elder Abuse Solutions,
Weill Cornell Medicine
New York, NY, USA

ISBN 978-3-031-97783-1 ISBN 978-3-031-97784-8 (eBook)
https://doi.org/10.1007/978-3-031-97784-8

This Springer imprint is published by the registered company Springer Nature Switzerland AG
The registered company address is: Gewerbestrasse 11, 6330 Cham, Switzerland

This book is dedicated to Adult Protective Services workers across the country. Their tireless work with adults in need of their services has been an inspiration to these authors.

Introduction

The impetus for this book was to bring to the reader the experiences of the authors who have participated on multidisciplinary elder abuse teams for the past decade. Elder abuse is an emerging field that will require more professionals to become adept at working in this area. Identification of the indicators of the abuse is complicated, nuanced, and requires the expertise of multiple professionals.

The cases presented throughout this book are representative of the complex, challenging issues front-line elder abuse service workers face every day. The book and its recommendations are by no means meant to be prescriptive, all encompassing, or the opinion of all. Each case of abuse and neglect is as unique as the victim and their circumstances.

We hope that the content will be useful as a guide for professionals who are working with elder abuse and neglect victims. We have intentionally kept recommendations general as availability of services, legal statutes, and regulations vary greatly across the country. However, in the authors' experience, the basic components of elder abuse cases carries across state lines and the interventions are comparable from coast to coast.

Elder abuse victims are among the most vulnerable of older adults. Their stories and experiences are often overlooked and minimized. Ageism has rendered older adults less valuable in our society. We encourage the reader to hear the voice of the victim in each chapter—to appreciate their unique situations, cultural concerns, and individual wishes.

Our hope is that the readers will utilize this book as a guide to begin their exploration into learning more about elder abuse. Utilizing emerging tools such as Artificial Intelligence, technical ways of connecting and social media can help to enhance our learning, recognition of elder abuse, and ultimately greatly diminish risks of abuse to vulnerable older adults.

Acknowledgments

Thank you to Erin Barry, Michael Roth, Jane Sarnoff, and Susan Shulman for proofreading, editing, and reference checks. Thank you to our families, friends, and colleagues who gave us encouragement and love during the process. We acknowledge the older adults who have suffered abuse, neglect, mistreatment, and financial exploitations. We hope this book will help inform emerging professionals about the experiences of older adult victims and more effectively intervene to help them live safe and productive lives.

The original version of the book has been revised. A correction to this book can be found at https://doi.org/10.1007/978-3-031-97784-8_12

Contents

Contributors

Robert Abrams (Retired) Department of Psychiatry, Weill Cornell Medicine, New York, NY, USA

Cynthia Amodeo Barrier Free Living, Bronx, NY, USA

Georgia J. Anetzberger Schools of Applied Social Sciences and Medicine, Case Western Reserve University and Consultant in Private Practice, South Euclid, OH, USA

Elizabeth M. Bloemen Division of Geriatrics, University of Colorado School of Medicine, Aurora, CO, USA

Alyssa Elman VEPT Supervising Social Worker, Weill Cornell Medicine, New York, NY, USA

Lisa Gibbs Division of Geriatric Medicine and Gerontology, Department of Family Medicine, University of California, Irvine, CA, USA

Jacqueline S. Gray The Native Center for Behavioral Health, University of Iowa College of Public Health, Iowa City, IA, USA

Candace Heisler Assistant District Attorney, San Francisco, San Francisco, CA, USA (Retired)
Heisler and Associates, San Bruno, CA, USA

Mark Lachs Division of Geriatrics and Palliative Medicine, Weill Cornell Medicine, New York, NY, USA

Veronica LoFaso (Retired) Division of Geriatrics and Palliative Medicine, Weill Cornell Medicine, New York, NY, USA

Richard Machemer (Retired) St. John Fisher University, Rochester, NY, USA

Arlene Markarian Safe Observant Seniors Program, FCA-Family and Children's Center, Garden City, NY, USA

Nancy Needell Psychiatry, Weill Cornell Medicine, New York, NY, USA

Marlena Orme Burke Rehabilitation Center, White Plains, NY, USA

Dina Patel Gramercy Psychiatry and Weill Cornell Medicine, New York, NY, USA

Lisa Rachmuth Division of Geriatrics and Palliative Medicine, Center for Elder Abuse Solutions, Weill Cornell Medicine, New York, NY, USA

Geoffrey Rogers The Learning and Development Projects at the Silberman School of Social Work, Hunter College, City University of New York, New York, NY, USA

Tony Rosen Vulnerable Elder Protection Team, Weill Cornell Medicine/New York-Presbyterian Hospital, New York, NY, USA

Karen Webber Skuse CPA, CFE Founder, Fraudfindr, Rochester, NY, USA

Elaine Suben The Center on Aging, NY Presbyterian Hospital, New York, NY, USA

Pamela B. Teaster Center for Gerontology, Virginia Tech, Blacksburg, VA, USA

Sarah Tietz Division of Geriatrics, University of Colorado School of Medicine, Aurora, CO, USA

Page Ulrey Elder Abuse Unit, King County Prosecuting Attorney's Office, Seattle, WA, USA

Kathy Van Olst District Attorney's Office, Seattle, WA, USA

Chapter 1
Elder Abuse: An Overview

Georgia J. Anetzberger

Origins and Early Depictions

Situations of elder abuse have been depicted in legend, literature, and historical account for hundreds of years [1, 2]. Nevertheless, recognition of elder abuse as a problem, worthy of public attention and resolution, only goes back about 70 years, with two notable points of origin.

The earliest point of origin occurred during the mid-1950s and 1960s with conversations in urban centers, like Cleveland and San Diego, about the growing number of older adults, often impaired and sometimes mentally or cognitively disabled, left behind as younger family members moved away in search of better jobs and more opportunity in an era of prosperity and growth. Community leaders in such centers were worried that these older adults might succumb to self-neglect or exploitation without outside intervention. In the process they exchanged case studies to illuminate and provide evidence of their concerns. These included the situation of Mrs. Rudolph, who at "age 88, lived in her own apartment on a site scheduled for demolition [with] rubbish as well as spoiled food…contributing to vermin infestation…She was forgetful, frequently losing money or her key, distrustful [of outside help]" ([3], pp. 121–122). Case examples discussed also included the circumstances of "Mrs. S., a 77-year-old widow, living in her own home…a recluse, hasn't bathed in two years…In winter the furnace goes out and water pipes burst, so there is no heat or water, and Mrs. S. tries to heat the whole house with a kitchen burner" ([4], p. 50). Situations like these brought attention to the problem and set the stage for development of adult protective services (APS) as an intervention to assist older adults potentially subject to such harm. Although led by social workers, from the

G. J. Anetzberger (✉)
Schools of Applied Social Sciences and Medicine, Case Western Reserve University and Consultant in Private Practice, South Euclid, OH, USA
e-mail: gia@case.edu

V. LoFaso, L. Rachmuth (eds.), *Elder Abuse and Neglect*,
https://doi.org/10.1007/978-3-031-97784-8_1

beginning APS was seen as needing the expertise and assistance of multiple other professionals, particularly physicians and attorneys [5].

The second point of origin for elder abuse began in the mid-1970s as physicians in both the United States and Great Britain drew attention to other potential harms inflicted on older adults, particularly physical abuse. Butler [6] describes a "67-year-old woman, widowed eight years, [who] was regularly beaten up by her 35-year-old unmarried son. She had turned her little money and her property over to the son. He stopped working". Burston [7] labels as "granny-battering" instances he observed and could confirm as a hospital physician, noting "that elderly patients have been battered by relatives before admission to hospital and in which there has been no doubt that the battering was deliberate". Social workers heard this alarm call from physicians and initiated research on elder abuse just a few years later. At conferences continents apart, they presented their findings. Lau and Kosberg [8] had identified 39 cases of elder abuse among the 404 older adults served by Cleveland's Chronic Illness Center during the past year, with three-fourths having been physically abused and over half psychologically abused. Of the eight forms of abuse identified, nearly two-thirds of the clients suffered from multiple (poly-victimization), with the typical perpetrator being the adult child of the victim. In contrast, Rathbone-McCuan [9] spent several years gathering case material from practicing clinicians whose older adult clients exhibited evidence of non-accidental physical abuse or physically endangering neglect. Ten such cases were identified. Of these, nearly all of the older adults had been repeatedly struck or kicked by adult children; As a result of her husband's neglect, she lay comatose with bed sores covering her body.

Although physicians and social workers may have led in elder abuse recognition and response, more recently the field has attracted other professionals. These have included those in law enforcement, such as police officers and prosecutors, notably present beginning the last two decades of the twentieth century, when the problem was increasingly seen as a crime to be punished. Also included during the first two decades of the twenty-first century have been those in finance, such as forensic accountants and investment advisors, where everything from improprieties in asset management to family theft inflicted on older adults has become a matter of concern and increasing attention. Payne and Strasser [10] offer a series of case studies which capture both professional approaches, including a caregiver who misappropriated tens of thousands of dollars from an older adult client who was deaf, blind, and wheelchair bound (cited by the National Association of Attorney Generals).

Definition and Forms

There is broad agreement that causing or attempting to cause harm to an older adult is a problem. There is less agreement about what to call it or how the problem should be defined. Elder abuse was the first used terminology. It also is the most familiar and accepted. The National Center on Elder Abuse categorizes elder abuse as, included under this umbrella, seven distinct forms, namely abandonment, emotional or psychological abuse, financial abuse or exploitation, neglect, physical abuse, self-neglect, and sexual abuse. Additional forms have been recognized by other sources, including confinement and undue influence by the Office for Victims of Crime [11] and violation of rights by the Long-Term Care Ombudsman Program [12]. Still other forms reflect attempts to nuance the concept of elder abuse, with divisions by setting or perpetrator intent.

However, elder abuse is not the only concept employed when discussing the problem of harm perpetrated against an older adult. Others include elder mistreatment, elder maltreatment, and abuse in later life. Descriptors used in distinguishing these concepts include those related to the act, the type of relationship between the victim and perpetrator, and the vulnerability of the victim. As a result, some concepts are seen as more expansive than others. Specifically, elder abuse tends to have the broadest definition, covering the most forms of harm, settings for its occurrence, and potential perpetrators. In contrast, abuse in later life has the narrowest focus, covering only those victims and abusers having close interpersonal involvement who reside in the community. It also covers fewer forms of harm, typically those associated with intimate partner violence. Elder mistreatment usually requires that victim and perpetrator be in a trusted relationship (which elder abuse does not), and unlike elder mistreatment, elder maltreatment includes self-neglect among its covered forms (which elder abuse does as well).

Defining elder abuse has never been easy. Understanding what it means has changed as the field of study evolved, professional groups interested in it were added, and debates occurred over such varied features as the necessary relationship between victim and perpetrator. It can be said that we are closer to agreement, but not quite there.

Present Understanding

Theory As applied to elder abuse, theory represents how the problem is conceptualized or viewed. It helps to identify patterns, explain change, and enlighten future directions. It also frames the way research is conducted and analyzed. The need for theories or conceptual models to understand, inform, or drive elder abuse was recognized during the late 1970s. In a presentation at the Annual Scientific Meeting of the Gerontological Society of America, Kosberg [13] suggested that several theories used for other abused populations, particularly children and intimate partners, may have relevance for elder abuse, including conflict, social structural and ecological theories.

Unfortunately, progress in elder abuse theory development proved to be so slow that 30 plus years after Kosberg's presentation, the National Institute of Justice [14] felt the need to convene a meeting of elder abuse researchers to discuss the matter.

The meeting kicked off with recognition that "elder abuse research tends to be light on or devoid of theory" and there is urgency to identify "concrete ways to encourage the use of elder abuse theories". More than a decade later, there seems to be widespread consensus that we have made progress in recognizing the need for theory development and use. However, there remains little agreement on which theories should dominate and too much research that is devoid of theory. In addition, most theories applied to elder abuse are still borrowed from other fields, including those representing other abused populations, whose characteristics and circumstances may differ from those of abused older adults [15, 16].

Jackson [17] categorizes existing theories applied to elder abuse as interpersonal (e.g., caregiver stress, social exchange), socio-cultural (e.g., power and control, routine activities), or multisystem (e.g., bio-psychosocial, ecological). Among these categories, most elder abuse theories seem to be interpersonal in nature [18], although there is growing use of multisystem theories.

Prevalence and Incidence Elder abuse is more common than most Americans believe. Large scale studies of the problem suggest that, excluding self-neglect, the past year rate globally is 15.7% [19]. Studies in the United States present ranges from 7.6% to 11% for community-dwelling older adults, with emotional abuse, financial exploitation, and neglect more common than other forms [20–24]. In addition, the lifetime prevalence rate of 21% is almost double the highest for past year elder abuse, with 12% of Americans experiencing poly-victimization [25]. Less is known about the scope of self-neglect, largely due to fewer studies and methodological concerns regarding the ones that exist. However, from those available, the rate seems low, between 0.5 and 7 per 1000 older adults annually [26]. Finally, since elder abuse incidence and prevalence studies typically exclude older adults with dementia and those in residential care facilities, it is worth noting that research on these populations suggests that elder abuse occurrence tends to be greater, perhaps as high as one in two for older adults with dementia [27, 28] and two in three for facility staff admitting to the commission of past year abuse, with psychological abuse more than twice as common as the next most reported form by residents [29]. Moreover, the rates of all types of elder abuse tend to be greater in nursing homes than other care settings, including assisted living and home care [30], with some evidence to suggest that reports of abuse cases in nursing homes tends to be on the rise [31].

Elder abuse is far more common than reports of it would suggest, despite mandatory reporting laws in all states but New York. Each decade since the 1980s seems to produce a new study exploring the number of elder abuse situations that come to public attention. However, comparisons among the studies are difficult, since the methods, populations, and even relevant local policy shows notable variation [22, 32, 33]. The most recent such study, focused on New York State, found that only one in 24 incidents of various elder abuse forms was reported, falling to one in 44 for financial exploitation and even lower to one in 57 for neglect [22]. Among professionals required to report elder abuse, social workers and law enforcement personnel tend to be most likely, and physicians the least likely to do so (e.g., [22, 34]).

Reasons given for non-reporting include concern that reporting could further endanger the victim and belief that the agency charged with responding may not do so either promptly or effectively [35, 36].

Risk and Protective Factors There are characteristics or conditions which have been found through research to increase (risk factors) or decrease (protective factors) the occurrence of elder abuse. In general, risk factors and protective factors can be organized under one or more of three possible entities, namely the victim, perpetrator, or context bringing the victim and perpetrator together. Although other entities have been noted, such as environment, culture, or community, they have been little investigated.

It is widely understood that the larger the number and longer the exposure of risk factors, the greater will be the likelihood of elder abuse occurrence. Conversely, the larger the number and longer the exposure of protective factors, the less likely it is that elder abuse will happen. Identifying risk and protective factors is important for elder abuse prevention, detection, and assessment. However, research to date has been significant with respect to risk factors and minimal on protective factors. Therefore, our understanding of these matters is decidedly uneven.

The many studies and reports of elder abuse risk factors reflect various methods and professional perspectives, sometimes making comparisons difficult (e.g., [17, 37–41]). Nonetheless, overall the most commonly identified risk factors include:

- Victim: cognitive impairment or dementia, poor physical health or frailty, functional dependence, lack of social support, and problem behaviors. (Others often named include low income, past abuse, substance abuse, and recent losses.)
- Perpetrator: substance abuse, mental health disorders, financial or housing dependence on the victim, behavioral problems (such as antisocial behavior or hostility), past history of violence, prior criminal record, and social isolation. (Additional perpetrator risk factors often are specific to persons assuming the role of caregiver, including a reluctance to take on that role, inexperience in doing it, lack of empathy for the care recipient, and history of childhood victimization.)
- Context for bringing victim and perpetrator together: shared living arrangements, lack of social supports, stress from external factors, and history of family disharmony.

Finally, the literature on risk factors also suggests some variation by form of elder abuse. For example, lack of social support, functional dependence, and past trauma have been found associated with emotional abuse, and poor physical health, cognitive impairment, mental health disorders, and lack of social supports with self-neglect.

The very limited research on protective factors to elder abuse suggests that characteristics or conditions on the part of the victim, like social support and strong community networks, can reduce problem occurrence (National Center on Elder Abuse, n.d.b). Where research is greater, namely with respect to financial exploitation, identified protective factors tend to be more numerous and include having a partner, financial literacy, established routines, positive outlook on life, and knowledge about how to report the problem [17, 42–45].

Effects Effects are the harmful outcomes of elder abuse. Generally speaking, they are experienced by victims. However, their reach can be more expansive, taking in family or friends and even society as a whole. Effects can be classified as signs, consequences, and costs.

Signs represent evidence of elder abuse infliction on victims. They are indicators or markers of its occurrence. Examples include bruising or wounds from physical abuse as well as malnutrition or dehydration from neglect. The detection of elder abuse signs has been aided by the development and use of screening and assessment tools. Some such tools are specific to the form of abuse, relationship of the perpetrator to the victim, or otherwise. Some also have been more rigorously tested than others [46, 47]. Indeed, the several systematic or scoping reviews on such tools suggest that further testing is much needed, especially with respect to validity and reliability on how and when the tools are to be used, with particular urgency on the need to evaluate them against measurable violence or health outcomes (e.g., [48–50]). Cautions like these have resulted in the US Prevention Services Task Force [51] failing to recommend universal screening of elder abuse, finding that "current evidence is insufficient to assess the balance of benefits and harms of screening". On the other hand, the American Medical Association and select other health care organizations recommend screening of all older patients for elder abuse. As an aid to deciding whether or not to screen, the National Center on Elder Abuse offers a Research to Practice Brief that examines the use of screening tools across various health care settings, pointing out both their potential benefits and potential harms [52].

Consequences represent the harmful outcomes of elder abuse. Unlike signs, they may not be evident through sensory perception. Podnieks and Thomas [53] classify consequences threefold as higher mortality, severe physical or emotional suffering, and more hospitalization and institutionalization. Higher mortality risk has been identified as the most credible of all elder abuse consequences [54]. Indeed, research on the subject has revealed that victims of self-neglect are two to six times and victims of other elder abuse forms two to three times more likely to die sooner than non-victims (e.g., [55, 56]). On the other hand, a recent New York state investigation found no difference in death rates between victims and non-victims over a 10-year period [57].

Finally, costs reflect financial loss from elder abuse. Generally, costs apply to victims and the monetary effect of financial exploitation or fraud. However, sometimes losses are calculated in other ways, such as (1) the cost to society of hospitalization, social services, and other interventions used to address elder abuse situations, and/or (2) the cost of lost opportunities or contributions for victims or others as a result of elder abuse infliction, such as through the inability to work or volunteer. Indeed, the cost of financial exploitation for victims is significant whether examined at the state or national level, and notwithstanding the methodology employed. For example, it is estimated that in one year, older adult victims lost $339 million in Utah [58] and between $174.7 and $451.5 million in Maine [59]. Nationally annual estimates range from $2.9 billion [60] to $36.48 billion [61].

Current Responses

Service Systems Given the complex nature and considerable scope of elder abuse, it should not be surprising that multiple service systems exist to respond to the problem. Each major service system is described below, with primary attention given to its purpose and activities.

Adult Protective Services represents the only system exclusively focused on addressing elder abuse (and usually the abuse of vulnerable younger adults as well). Anchored in state law and administrative policy (both of which show variation across the country), it typically operates out of public departments of social services or state units on aging. During the past decade federal government guidance has increased, particularly as a result of the Administration for Community Living providing a "home" for APS, with funding available to state programs during the recent pandemic and as part of its general budget for the first time in 2024. Throughout the country, the role of APS is to receive and investigate reports of abuse, neglect, and exploitation; evaluate client status and service needs; arrange or provide services to address harm and to prevent its reoccurrence; and work with other systems to seek legal intervention, if required, such as criminal penalty for perpetrators or surrogate or supportive decision-making for cognitively or mentally incapacitated victims. Because APS operates on the basis of self-determination, it means that clients able to make decisions can refuse the investigation or services offered. However, state statute offers APS the option of seeking through the courts involuntary intervention under proscribed circumstances, typically when the victim lacks decision-making capacity or is in emergency circumstances.

The Aging Network originated in 1965 with passage of the Older Americans Act (OAA). It has evolved ever since, with reauthorizations enabling it to be responsive to the changing needs and concerns of older adults nationwide. Elder abuse prevention became a designated activity in 1987, with the Long-Term Care Ombudsman Program (LTCO) being established almost a decade earlier to protect the rights (including the right to be free of elder abuse) of those older adults in nursing homes, later expanded to other residential care facilities and community-based long-term services and supports. In 1992 Title VII was enacted, combining and expanding elder rights and protection activities, which is done primarily through authorized formula grants to states and territories via their units on aging. Currently the grants support efforts to prevent elder abuse (such as through outreach, education, and exploring new prevention or intervention models), the LTCO, state legal assistance directed programs, and sometimes victim assistance activities. In addition, some OAA services can enable older adults to better manage on their own and therefore potentially prevent elder abuse occurrence (e.g., nutrition programs, transportation) or help caregivers better handle that role and prevent elder abuse infliction (e.g., respite care, counseling). Programs like these are usually available through area agencies on aging, county or municipal offices on aging, senior centers, and other community service organizations.

Domestic violence and sexual assault programs exist to insure the safety of abuse victims while holding their perpetrators accountable. That includes victims of abuse in later life, although not all such programs around the country have made special accommodations to serve this population. Typical available services include hotlines, information and referral, legal advocacy, emergency shelters, transitional housing, counseling, and support groups. Attention to older abused women first drew national attention in 1992 when AARP convened a forum on the needs of this group, ultimately producing a document on the subject and a directory of available services. Funding from various federal sources (e.g., Victims of Crime Act, Family Violence Prevention and Services Act, and Violence Against Women Act) enabled demonstration projects to address some of these needs and led to the establishment of the National Clearinghouse on Abuse in Later Life, which has as its purpose to offer related policy information, advocacy, and training or education.

Health care's interest in elder abuse has been slow to evolve, notwithstanding the fact that physicians were the first to bring the problem to national, indeed international, attention. This is unfortunate, because health care is vital to nearly every aspect of addressing elder abuse, from its detection and referral for investigation to its treatment of inflicted harm and risk factors that can contribute to harm occurrence. Health care settings include practitioner offices, clinics, hospitals, rehabilitation facilities, and mental health and substance abuse centers. Public policy on elder abuse and health care also has been minimal, outside of state mandatory reporting laws that include health care professionals, like physicians and nurses, more often than others. In addition, the US Centers for Disease Prevention and Control has provided uniform definitions and data elements for collecting data on elder abuse within a public health framework. Finally, select health care academic centers, like those at Cornell University and the University of Southern California, have become leaders in elder abuse research, undertaking studies to better understand the problem's etiology as well as ways to effectively screen for and treat it.

Law enforcement has as its purpose to address violations of the legal code, which include assault, theft, or domestic violence. In many states elder abuse itself is treated as one or more distinct crimes, and/or there may be an enhanced penalty when the crime victim is an older adult. Representatives of law enforcement are found in such settings as police stations, sheriff's departments, prosecutor offices, and courts. Law enforcement can investigate elder abuse as a crime, with the authority to arrest and prosecute perpetrators. Victim assistance programs cooperate with law enforcement, providing older adult crime victims with such services as counseling, court accompaniment, and information on victim compensation. On the civil side, law enforcement can execute protective or restraining orders, attempt to recover financial losses due to exploitation, seek compensation for harm infliction, or enable the use of guardianship, civil commitment, or protective orders. Moreover, law enforcement is often the first responder in crisis situations (such as extreme self-neglect or severe physical abuse) and involved in well-being checks of vulnerable or impaired older adults. In some locales, specialized units for elder abuse investigation or prosecution have been formed, such as in San Francisco and Seattle. Finally, the Elder Abuse Prevention and Prosecution Act, passed in 2017, requires the US Department of Justice to better prevent crimes against older adults through such provisions as authorizing each federal judicial district to designate an elder justice coordinator and the Federal Bureau of Investigation to provide comprehensive elder abuse training for agents.

Interventions Besides service systems, interventions exist which have as their purpose either preventing the occurrence of elder abuse or addressing damage caused by its infliction. More specifically, interventions represent assorted programs and practices. If their purpose is prevention, then they attempt to eliminate or reduce identified risk factors. If their purpose is treatment, then they address the effects of elder abuse.

The importance of elder abuse prevention has a long history, acknowledged by some of the field's first researchers (e.g., [62, 63]). Nonetheless, there was early recognition that attention given to preventing the problem was much less than that extended to response once it had occurred [64]. More than 30 years later that conclusion still stands [65, 66]. Equally as discouraging, there have been multiple systematic reviews on elder abuse prevention measures which collectively suggest that there is little quality research attesting to their effectiveness and worth (e.g., [67–69]). Not surprisingly, Stein [70] concludes, "As a summary statement, the field lacks systematic and methodologically sound studies to measure and evaluate the long-term impacts of indicated prevention interventions". Promising practices in the area of elder abuse prevention often aim at providing caregivers with supports (e.g., respite, counseling) or improving their knowledge or attitudes (e.g., interactive groups, training). However, once again there is minimal evidence of their value at stopping elder abuse. In addition, although some such measures have been developed specifically for elder abuse (e.g., Take AIM Against Elder Abuse Intervention Prevention Model), most were developed for other purposes and simply came to be used to address elder abuse as well.

Although there are more measures to treat elder abuse than prevent it, by and large, once again they usually have been borrowed from other fields, such as child abuse or intimate partner violence, or developed for other purposes [17, 71]. The latter is illustrated through services offered by the Aging Network that can assist victims but were not developed specifically for them, like senior centers, nutrition programs, personal care, and transportation [72]. Most interventions actually developed to treat elder abuse target either physical abuse or financial exploitation. In addition, rarely are treatments developed for perpetrators, despite some evidence that they may be more likely to accept and benefit from such assistance [73]. Further, there is indication that select treatments may actually increase rates of abuse occurrence [74]. Finally, and perhaps most discouraging, is the simple lack of evidence for nearly all existing treatments [68, 75, 76].

Multidisciplinary Approaches This chapter ends much as it began, with recognition that it takes more than any single professional discipline to address elder abuse. Because of the problem's complexity and challenges, multiple disciplines, working together, are required to understand its many dimensions and provide the diversity of interventions that might be needed [77]. As we saw with the onset of APS more than a half century ago, the essential disciplines seem to be social services, medicine, and law. However, others, from animal rescue to finance, may be required for their particular expertise or resources, depending on the form of elder abuse or the dynamics of the individual situation being addressed.

Multiple professional disciplines can coalesce informally for collective action or case handling around elder abuse. This happens naturally all of the time. However, the field is noteworthy for its formation and use of various multidisciplinary networks and teams, which offer more sustained and structured support [78–80]. Such networks and teams can form at either the state or local level. In addition, some purposefully are time-limited and others are ongoing, depending on their particular aims and levels of commitment.

Networks have as their function to collaborate across systems and disciplines in order to improve elder abuse detection, prevention, and treatment through policy, practice, or education initiatives. Examples include coalitions, summits, task forces, or advisory councils. Networks also can serve to create and support teams. Teams represent assemblies of professionals across disciplines and systems for the function of case review and recommendation. Some teams are general in their case focus, willing to consider any and all forms and situations of elder abuse. Others are specialized, focused on a single form or situation, such as financial abuse or hoarding. Examples include community case consult teams, adult protection teams, financial abuse specialist teams, fatality review teams, and forensic center teams.

Research on the effectiveness of networks and teams is limited, except perhaps for forensic center teams (e.g., [81, 82]). However, their popularity is widespread, evidenced in the mapping of several hundred by the US Department of Justice and most recently through federal funding that established the National Center for State and Tribal Elder Justice Coalitions in 2022 for the purpose of providing guidance and support to create and sustain state and tribal coalitions which address elder abuse and other elder justice issues.

References

1. Reinharz S. Loving and hating one's elders: twin themes in legend and literature. In: Pillemer KA, Wolf RS, editors. Elder abuse: conflict in the family. Auburn House: Dover; 1986. p. 25–48.
2. Stearns PJ. Old age family conflict: the perspective of the past. In: Pillemer KA, Wolf RS, editors. Elder abuse: conflict in the family. Auburn House: Dover; 1986. p. 3–24.
3. O'Neill V. Protecting older people. Public Welf. 1965;23(2):119–27.
4. Ross HA. Protective services for adults. Gerontologist. 1968;8(1):50–3.

5. Hall GH. Protective services for adults. In: Morris R, editors. Encyclopedia of social work. 16th ed. 1971 pp. 999, 1002–6.
6. Butler RN. Being old in America. New York: Harper Row; 1975.
7. Burston GR. Granny-battering. BNJ Med. 1975;3:592.
8. Lau EE, Kosberg JI. Abuse of the elderly by informal care providers: practice and research issues. Paper presented at the Gerontological Society of America 31st annual meeting, Dallas, TX, November 1978. 1978.
9. Rathbone-McCuan E. Intergenerational family violence and neglect: the aged as victims of reactivated and reverse neglect. Paper presented at the 11th international congress of gerontology, Tokyo, 20–25 August 1978. 1978.
10. Payne BK, Strasser SM. Financial exploitation of older persons in adult care settings: comparisons to physical abuse and the justice system's response. J Eld Abuse Neg. 2012;24:231–50.
11. Office for Victims of Crime, Training and Technical Assistance Center. Elder abuse. 2012.
12. Administration for Community Living. The long-term care Ombudsman Program: protecting the rights of residents. 2019.
13. Kosberg JI. Family conflict and abuse of the elderly: theoretical and methodological issues. Paper presented at the annual scientific meeting of the Gerontological Society of America, Washington, DC, November 1979; 1979.
14. National Institute of Justice. Elder mistreatment: using theory in research: meeting summary. 2014.
15. Anetzberger GJ, Podnieks E, et al. Elder abuse in The United States of America. In: Teaster PB, Anetzberger GJ, et al., editors. The worldwide face of elder abuse. Cham: Springer; 2023. p. 125–43.
16. Roberto KA, Teaster PB. Theorizing elder abuse. In: Dong X, editor. Elder abuse: research, practice and policy. Cham: Springer; 2017. p. 21–41.
17. Jackson SL. Understanding elder abuse: a clinician's guide. Washington DC: American Psychological Association; 2018.
18. Burnight K, Mosqueda L. Theoretical model development in elder mistreatment. Washington DC: National Institute of Justice; 2011.
19. Yon Y, Mikton C, et al. Elder abuse prevalence in community settings: a systematic review and meta-analysis. Lancet Glob Health. 2017;5:e147–56.
20. Acierno R, Hernandez MA, et al. Prevalence and correlates of emotional, physical, sexual, and financial abuse and potential neglect in the United States. The National Elder Mistreatment Study. Am J Public Health. 2010;100(2):292–7.
21. Kudon HZ, Herbst JH, et al. Prevalence estimates and factors associated with violence among older adults: National Intimate Partner and Sexual Violence (NISVS) Survey, 2016/2017. J Eld Abuse Neg. 2024;36(1):67–88.
22. Lachs M, Berman J. Under the radar: New York state elder abuse prevalence study. Lifespan of Greater Rochester, Inc., Weill Cornell Medical Center of Cornell University, New York City Department of Aging; 2011.
23. Laumann EO, Leitsch SA, et al. Elder mistreatment in the United States: prevalence estimates from a nationally representative study. J Gerontol B Psychol Sci Soc Sci. 2008;63B(4):S248–54.
24. Rosay AB, Mulford CF. Prevalence estimates and correlates of elder abuse in the United States: the National Intimate Partner and sexual violence survey. J Eld Abuse Neg. 2017;29(1):1–14.
25. Wong JS, Breslau H, et al. The social relationship context of elder mistreatment. Gerontologist. 2020;60(6):1029–39.
26. Dyer CB, Reyes-Ortiz CA. Epidemiology of elder self-neglect. In: Dong X, editor. Elder abuse: research, practice and policy. Cham: Springer; 2017. p. 125–39.
27. Moqueda L, Burnight K, et al. The abuse intervention model: a pragmatic approach to intervention for elder mistreatment. J Am Geriatr Soc. 2016;64(9):1879–83.
28. Wiglesworth A, Mosqueda L, et al. Screening for abuse and neglect or people with dementia. J Am Geriatr Soc. 2010;58:493–7.

29. Yon Y, Mikton C, et al. The prevalence of self-reported elder abuse among older women in community settings: a systematic review and meta-analysis. TraumaViolence Abuse. 2019;20(2):245–59.
30. Page C, Conner T, et al. The effect of care setting on elder abuse results from a Michigan survey. J Eld Abuse Neg. 2009;21(3):239–52.
31. Mogaka EN, Bistas KG, et al. Elderly abuse and neglect in American nursing homes: a systematic review. Allegheny Health Sci J. 2020;2(1):20–34.
32. National Center on Elder Abuse & Westat Inc. The national elder abuse incidence study: final report. 1998.
33. Pillemer KA, Finkelhor D. The prevalence of elder abuse: a random sample survey. The Gerontologist. 1998;28(1):51–7.
34. Teaster P, Dugar T, et al. The 2004 survey of state adult protective services: abuse of adults 60 years of age and older. Washington, DC: National Center on Elder Abuse; 2006.
35. Jogerst GJ, Xu Y, et al. Iowa family physician's reporting of elder abuse: 20-year follow-up. J Eld Abuse Neg. 2024;36(1):25–40.
36. Miller CA. Elder abuse and nursing: what nurses need to know and can do about it. New York: Springer; 2017.
37. Chen R, Dong X. Risk factors of elder abuse. In: Dong X, editor. Elder abuse: research, practice and policy. Cham: Springer; 2017. p. 93–107.
38. Johannesen M, LoGiudice D. Elder abuse: a systematic review of risk factors in community dwelling elders. Age Ageing. 2013;42(3):292–8.
39. Miller CA, Anetzberger GJ. Elder abuse and neglect. In: Miller CA, editor. Nursing for wellness in older adults. 9th ed. Philadelphia: Wolters Kluwer; 2023. p. 166–96.
40. Pillemer K, Burnes D, et al. Elder abuse: global situation, risk factors, and prevention strategies. Gerontologist. 2016;56(Suppl-2):S194–205.
41. Storey JE. Risk factors for elder abuse and neglect: a review of the literature. Aggress Violent Behav. 2020;50:101339.
42. Hall L, Moray J, et al. Financial stressors and resources associated with financial exploitation. Innov Aging. 2022;6(2):1–10.
43. James BD, Boyle PA, et al. Correlates of susceptibility to scams in older adults without dementia. J Eld Abuse Neg. 2014;26:107–22.
44. Liu P-J, Wood S, et al. The role of social support in elder financial exploitation using a community sample. Innov Aging. 2017;1(1):igx016.
45. Shao J, Zhang Q, et al. Why are older adult victims of fraud? Current knowledge and prospects regarding older adults' vulnerability to fraud. J Eld Abuse Neg. 2019;31(3):225–43.
46. Daly JM. Elder abuse prevention. University of Iowa College of Nursing; 2017.
47. Schofield MJ. Screening for elder abuse: tools and effectiveness. In: Dong X, editor. Elder abuse: research, practice and policy. Cham: Springer; 2017. p. 161–99.
48. Gallione C, Molin AD, et al. Screening tools for identification of elder abuse: a systematic review. J Med Clin Nurs. 2017;26(15–16):2154–76.
49. Santos-Rodrigues RC, Silva Brandão BML, et al. Assessment tools for elder abuse: scoping review. J School Nurs Univ San Paulo. 2022;56:e20220115.
50. Van Royen K, Royen PV, et al. Elder abuse assessment tools and interventions for use in the home environment: a scoping review. Clin Interv Aging. 2020;15:1793–807.
51. US Preventive Services Task Force. Intimate partner violence, elder abuse, and abuse of vulnerable adults: screening (Published final recommendations). 2018.
52. National Center on Elder Abuse. Research to practice: elder abuse screening tools for healthcare professionals. 2016.
53. Podnieks E, Thomas C. The consequences of elder abuse. In: Dong X, editor. Elder abuse: research, practice and policy. Cham: Springer; 2017. p. 109–23.
54. Yunus RM, Hairi NN, et al. Consequences of elder abuse and neglect: a systematic review of observational studies. Trauma Violence Abuse. 2019;20(2):197–213.

55. Dong X, Simon M, et al. Elder self-neglect and abuse and mortality risk in a community-dwelling population. JAMA. 2009;302(5):517–26.
56. Lachs MS, Williams CS, et al. The mortality of elder mistreatment. JAMA. 1998;280(5):428–32.
57. Pillemer K, Burnes D, et al. Lack of association of elder mistreatment with mortality. J Gerontol Ser A. 2022;77(8):1699–705.
58. Gunther J. The Utah cost of financial exploitation. Utah Division of Aging and Adult services and Bank of American Fork; 2010.
59. Griffin E, McGuire C, et al. Financial exploitation of Maine's older adults: an analysis of Maine adult protective services and legal services for the elderly case records, state fiscal years 2010–2016. University of Southern Maine, Cutler Institute of Health and Social Policy; 2017.
60. MetLife Mature Market Institute. The MetLife study of elder financial abuse: crimes of occasion, desperation, and predation against American elders. New York: Metropolitan Life Insurance Company; 2011.
61. True Link Financial. The True Link report on elder financial abuse. 2015.
62. Douglass RL. Opportunities for prevention of domestic neglect and abuse of the elderly. Prev Hum Serv. 1983;3(1):135–50.
63. Fulmer T. Overview of prevention research. Paper presented at the family violence research conference, University of New Hampshire, 11 July 1987. 1987.
64. Wolf RS. Strategies for the prevention of elder abuse. Paper presented at the annual conference of the American Society on Aging, Chicago, 9 March 1993. 1993.
65. National Center on Elder Abuse. Research brief: intervention in elder mistreatment. 2023a.
66. National Center on Elder Abuse. What is elder abuse? 2023b.
67. Baker PR, Francis DP, et al. Interventions for preventing elder abuse: applying findings of a new Cochrane review. Age Aging. 2017;46:346–8.
68. Marshall K, Herbst J, et al. Do interventions to prevent or stop abuse and neglect among older adults work? A systematic review of reviews. J Eld Abuse Neg. 2020;32(5):409–33.
69. Pillemer KA, Mueller-Johnson KU, et al. Interventions to prevent elder mistreatment. In: Doll LS, Bonzo SE, et al., editors. Handbook of injury and violence prevention. New York: Springer; 2007. p. 241–54.
70. Stein K. Elder abuse prevention interventions. In: Dong X, editor. Elder abuse: research, practice and policy. Cham: Springer; 2017. p. 433–57.
71. Chalk R, King PA. Violence in families: assessing prevention and treatment programs. Washington DC: National Academies Press; 1998.
72. Yonashiro-Cho J, Meyer K, et al. The aging network. In: Dong X, editor. Elder abuse: research, practice and policy. Cham: Springer; 2017. p. 297–315.
73. Nahmiash D, Reis M. Most successful intervention strategies for abused older adults. J Eld Abuse Neg. 2000;12(3/4):53–70.
74. Ploeg J, Fear J, et al. A systematic review of interventions for elder abuse. J Eld Abuse Neg. 2009;27(3):187–210.
75. Burnes D, MacNeil A, et al. A scoping review of outcomes in elder abuse intervention research: the current landscape and where to go next. Aggress Violent Behav. 2021;57:101476.
76. Rosen T, Elman A, et al. Review of programs to combat elder mistreatment: focus on hospitals and level of resources needed. J Am Geriatr Soc. 2019;67(6):1286–94.
77. Nerenberg L. Elder abuse prevention: emerging trends and promising practices. New York: Springer; 2008.
78. Anetzberger GJ. Elder abuse multidisciplinary teams. In: Dong X, editor. Elder abuse: research, practice and policy. Cham: Springer; 2017. p. 417–32.
79. Anetzberger GJ. The evolution of a multidisciplinary response to elder abuse. Marquette Elder's Advisor. 2011;13(1):107–28.
80. Galdamez G, Avent E, et al. Elder abuse multidisciplinary teams and networks: understanding national intervention approaches. Innov Aging. 2018;2(Suppl 1):763.

81. Gassoumis ZD, Navarro AE, et al. Protecting victims of elder financial exploitation: the role of an elder abuse forensic center in referring victims for conservatorship. J Ment Health Aging. 2015;19(9):790–8.
82. Navarro AE, Gassoumis ZD, et al. Holding abusers accountable: an elder abuse forensic center increases criminal prosecution of financial exploitation. Gerontologist. 2013;53(2):303–12.

Chapter 2
Physical Abuse

Candace Heisler, Alyssa Elman, and Tony Rosen

Introduction

Though elder mistreatment is common and has serious consequences, it is often not identified or reported to the authorities [1–4]. It includes physical abuse, sexual abuse, verbal and psychological abuse, neglect, and financial exploitation [1, 2, 4]. The focus of this chapter is physical abuse, which is typically defined as "the intentional use of physical force that may result in bodily injury, physical pain, or impairment." [5] Examples include slapping, kicking, pushing, pulling hair, burning, strangling, using objects as weapons, using firearms and/or knives, as well as using physical restraints and force-feeding [5].

Though physical abuse occurs less frequently than other forms of mistreatment, with a prevalence of 0.2–2.1% among community-dwelling older adults, it can be particularly devastating [1, 6–8]. Physical abuse may occur within a caregiving relationship or in the context of domestic abuse, family violence, or sexual violence [9].

C. Heisler
Assistant District Attorney, San Francisco, San Francisco, CA, USA (Retired)

Heisler and Associates, San Bruno, CA, USA

A. Elman
VEPT Supervising Social Worker, Weill Cornell Medicine, New York, NY, USA

T. Rosen (✉)
Vulnerable Elder Protection Team, Weill Cornell Medicine/New York-Presbyterian Hospital, New York, NY, USA
e-mail: aer2006@med.cornell.edu

V. LoFaso, L. Rachmuth (eds.), *Elder Abuse and Neglect*,
https://doi.org/10.1007/978-3-031-97784-8_2

Unlike other types of mistreatment, typical victims do not often have substantial physical or cognitive impairment [9]. Some risk factors for becoming a victim include social isolation, low socioeconomic status, poor mental health, history of family violence, traumatic event exposure, and substance abuse [1, 8, 10]. Risk factors for perpetrators are mental illness, substance abuse, caregiver stress, history of family violence, and traumatic event exposure [1, 8, 10].

Case Presentation

Police were called to the home of Mary Johnson, age 78, by a neighbor who heard screaming and objects hitting the wall. On arrival, a neighbor told officers "her son is at it again." The neighbor reported often hearing screams coming from the Johnson residence resulting in numerous calls to police. On prior occasions the neighbor had seen Mary with bruises to her face. Mary had told the neighbor that her son sometimes loses his temper when he drinks and hits her.

Officers knocked on the door of the Johnson home and were greeted by James, age 53. He said his mother had tripped on the carpet earlier that evening and was currently sleeping. After officers insisted on seeing Mary, James reluctantly admitted them. Mary was in the kitchen slumped over the table. She initially seemed confused and had difficulty answering the officers' questions. Officers saw bruises on her left cheek and swelling to her right eye. She was hoarse and gasping for air as though having an asthma attack.

Officers had Mary transported to the emergency department of the nearby hospital. James followed her to the hospital and stayed by her bedside. Emergency Medical Technicians (EMTs) reported that Mary's blood pressure was 200/120 and she seemed to have difficulty breathing when they initially arrived on scene.

The medical team asked James to sit in the waiting area and then evaluated Mary. Once Mary knew that James could not hear her, she told the nurse that her son had attacked her when she told him she was concerned about his drinking. She said this was not the first time. She said James struck her face with his fist, pushed her against a living room wall, and then put his hands around her neck. She saw spots and believed she was about to die. She said she may have passed out as she ended up on the ground without any recollection of how she got there. The physician noted that Mary had bruises to her left zygoma region, petechiae in both eyes, scalp, and ears, and bruising around her neck. She also had bruises in various stages of healing on her upper extremities. She was hoarse and complained of a sore throat.

Mary said she loved her son but was afraid of him and did not want to return home if he was there. She is very worried about him and wants him to get help. Police arrested James.

Physical Abuse Overview

For Medical Professionals

Assessment

For healthcare professionals, identifying physical elder abuse requires considering it in the differential when treating purportedly unintentional injuries or noting physical findings suggesting previous injuries. When evaluating older adults with injuries, it is imperative to get a detailed description of the history, including: the cause of the injury; the mechanism, who was present; how it was handled; and how soon the older adult sought care after the injury [11]. Clinicians should also obtain a comprehensive medical and social history, including immediate factors that led to the presentation as well as an understanding of the patient's baseline functioning [11] Clinicians may also inquire about activities of daily living (ADLs) and home management of the older adult, including handling finances, cooking, cleaning, taking medications, hygiene, cognition, and overall care needs [12].

While it may be tempting to gather history from a caregiver if the older adult has cognitive impairment or there is a language barrier, when considering elder mistreatment and physical abuse specifically, it is important to interview the patient directly. This should be done without the older adult's caregiver present to ensure privacy and confidentiality. Research indicates that people with dementia can often reliably describe how an injury occurred [13, 14]. One study suggests that 7% of cognitively intact older adults in the Emergency Department report mistreatment when asked directly about it, so it is important to ensure that the patient is provided an opportunity to disclose [15]. If the individual speaks another language or uses alternative methods of communication, using professional interpretation services is preferable to relying on family, so that the patient can feel comfortable and safe discussing sensitive topics such as possible mistreatment. If the older adult is unable to provide a full history, additional information may be obtained from other sources including their outpatient providers, family, and homecare and community agencies [12].

It is also essential to conduct a thorough biopsychosocial assessment to get a better understanding of the older adult. Exploring their medical history, asking about prior abuse, and getting a sense of their functioning at home is critical. Providers should inquire about any risks in the home environment as well as potential barriers to necessary resources [16]. Though professionals may feel uncomfortable, it is important to ask patients about each individual abuse type. If providers do not ask, older adults may not disclose. Older adults may feel more comfortable having these types of sensitive conversations with social workers, who are particularly adept at creating safe spaces and therapeutic alliances. The Emergency Department Elder Mistreatment Assessment Tool (ED-EMATS) may assist social workers who are not comfortable or familiar with this type of assessment [17].

Speaking to an older adult's outpatient provider, if available, may also provide insight into their baseline functioning and dynamics with family and caregivers [11].

Injury Patterns

Identifying physical elder mistreatment is often challenging for professionals. Differentiating between inflicted and accidental injuries in older adults is difficult because of normal physiologic changes that occur with aging such as osteopenia, thinning of the skin, easy bruising, and the effects of medications commonly used, such as anticoagulants [18–22]. Forensic injury patterns highly specific for physical elder abuse have not yet been described, though suggestive injury patterns exist that may help professionals assessing injured older adults to distinguish between abuse from unintentional injury, such as an accidental fall (See Table 2.1).

In addition to examining areas of reported injuries or pain, it is critical to conduct a thorough head-to-toe examination. This includes a full skin and intra-oral examination, being sure to note any decubitus ulcerations, fingernail and toenail hygiene, and dental issues. It is important to keep in mind that no physical finding is diagnostic in isolation, though suspicion should increase if multiple signs are present [19, 23–25]. Findings suggestive of previous, healing injuries may also contribute to a suggestive pattern.

Research is ongoing to establish an evidence base to support the specificity of certain types of injures in physical elder abuse. A study that compared older adults who presented with an accidental fall with older adults who were confirmed victims of physical abuse found that the latter often had bruises that were large (>5 cm) and located on the face, lateral right arm, or posterior torso [14]. Research has also suggested that injuries sustained by physical elder mistreatment victims were often

Table 2.1 Injury patterns suspicious for potential physical elder abuse

Bruising in atypical locations (not over bony prominences/on lateral arms, back, face, ears, or neck)
Patterned injuries (bite marks or injury consistent with the shape of a belt buckle, fingertip, or other object)
Wrist or ankle lesions or scars (suggesting inappropriate restraint)
Burns (particularly stocking/glove pattern suggesting forced immersion or cigarette pattern)
Multiple fractures or bruises of different ages
Traumatic alopecia or scalp hematomas
Subconjunctival, vitreous or retinal ophthalmic haemorrhages
Intraoral soft tissue injuries
For Strangulation
Redness or ecchymoses on neck
Neck swelling
Neck tenderness
Laryngeal and subcutaneous neck crepitus
Facial or conjunctival petechiae
sPtosis, facial droop, unilateral weakness

Refs. [19, 23–25, 30]

found on the head, neck, and upper extremities [18, 26, 27]. Compared with the older adult population presenting to the Emergency Department with a fall, older adult abuse victims are more likely to have injuries to the left cheek/zygoma. Neck and ear injuries occur commonly in abuse but not in cases from an accidental fall [28]. In addition, they are more likely to have maxillofacial, dental, and neck injuries with no upper and lower extremity injuries, suggesting that the simultaneous presence and absence of injuries may be helpful in differentiating intentional from unintentional injuries in older adults [28].

Strangulation

Strangulation may be involved in physical elder abuse and should be carefully assessed ~~for~~ in all cases in which physical abuse is suspected. All victims should be asked about whether they were strangled, or choked, during the assault or if they felt as if they couldn't breathe because of pressure on their neck. Hoarseness, dysphonia or aphonia occurs in roughly half of strangulation cases [29]. Some victims may present with dysphagia, odynophagia, dyspnea, and/or stridor [30]. Any injuries in the neck area should prompt consideration. Also, facial petechiae may occur due to strangulation because of venous congestion [30]. These may disappear within 1 day, though, and also appear in other conditions [30]. Healthcare providers should be mindful that the absence of external injuries is common in strangulation. Despite this, the sequela can be serious or even fatal if not recognized, including carotid dissection and intracranial hemorrhage [23]. Given physiologic changes association with aging, comorbid conditions, and previous brain disease, older adults are especially susceptible to cerebral injury after strangulation [23]. This cerebral injury may present with stroke-like signs and symptoms suggesting vascular or nerve damage, including ptosis, facial droop, or unilateral weakness [29, 31]. Strangulation as a cause of death increases with victim's age [23, 32, 46]. Older women are more likely to die from strangulation than men of the same age [23, 32]. Because of ageist beliefs that strangulation does not happen to older adults, strangulation is discounted as a cause of injury in many cases.

Imaging Correlates

Diagnostic imaging plays a critical role in detecting child abuse but is only starting to be recognized as a tool to identify physical elder abuse. Potential imaging correlates exist including co-occurring old and new fractures, high-energy fractures in the case of a low-energy mechanism, distal ulnar diaphyseal fractures, and small bowel hematomas [33, 34]. Notably, a hyoid fracture without an explanatory mechanism may suggest strangulation [29]. Clinicians who are concerned about physical elder abuse may want to consider discussing with a radiologist whether the imaging findings are consistent with the purported mechanism. Medical teams may also want to consider additional imaging including maxillofacial computed tomography scans and chest radiographs, to evaluate for acute and chronic fractures; this is analogous to the skeletal survey routinely performed in potential victims of child abuse [35–37]. MRI's have been shown to be a helpful tool in cases of suspected strangulation revealing vascular, muscular and laryngeal trauma not obvious to the naked eye [49].

Laboratory Tests

Conducting laboratory tests may also help determine if elder mistreatment has occurred. These tests can help clinicians detect anemia as well as potential dehydration (an elevated BUN/creatinine ratio) or malnutrition (low albumin) [38]. As with physical injuries, multiple abnormal results is more concerning than a single one. Unusual bruising may be more concerning in the context of normal platelet levels and coagulation studies. Clinicians can also check prescription medication levels (e.g., serum levels of antiepileptic drugs, international normalized ratio for individuals on warfarin, thyroid-stimulation hormone for people on levothyroxine) when assessing for mistreatment. Low levels in someone who is dependent on a caregiver for medication administration may suggest intentional or unintentional withholding, whereas high levels may indicate an intentional or unintentional overdose [38]. The presence of drugs that have not been prescribed or illicit drugs could suggest poisoning [38]. As a result, clinicians may also want to consider the urine toxicology screen [38].

Documentation in the Medical Chart

Documentation in the medical chart should be detailed and accurate, as this information may be utilized in the legal system [39]. All physical findings should be described thoroughly, including injury size, location, stage of healing, and if it is consistent with the alleged mechanism [11]. If possible, obtain permission from the patient or surrogate decision maker to take photos of visible injuries for the medical record A protocol for injury documentation exists to provide guidance [40]. Direct quotes from the patient about their experience can help bolster the documentation.

Considering the older adult's immediate safety and minimizing the risk of re-victimization should be the priority. The support of hospital security or nursing management may be required if the perpetrator is at bedside or there are concerns about the perpetrator coming to the hospital [11]. This is especially true if this individual is interfering with care. It can be necessary to restrict visitation or communication, provide a security watch, change the patients name, and/or notify local law enforcement. ED and hospital administration and legal may also be helpful in navigating challenging cases, such as when the suspected perpetrator is also the patient's health care decision-maker [11]. Providers with concerns for the patient's safety may want to facilitate an alternate living situation for the patient or consider an admission to the hospital [11]. Medical providers may exercise HIPAA exemptions in instances where there are concerns about the surrogate decision makers involvement in perpetrating the abuse (available at www.hhs.gov/ocr/privacy/hipaa/understanding).

Management and Referrals

For patients who will be discharged to the community from the ED or sent home from an outpatient visit, it is also important to consider how to address post-discharge unmet needs, safety, and well-being. Referrals to providers and services that can allow for continued supervision of the patient and reduce social isolation should be considered. Referrals can include a follow-up appointment with a primary care provider, setting up medication delivery, or facilitating safety visits by the police. Online tools such as www.findhelp.org can be used to find available social services by zip code. This may be especially useful if social workers or care managers are not present, such as in smaller EDs or during nights and weekends. In addition to providing resources and referrals, the ED providers help the older adult develop a safety plan, should the situation escalate again, which is instrumental in preventing future incidents. All older adults should be informed that they can return to the ED if they have safety concerns following discharge.

Mandatory Reporting

It is critical that clinical professionals who work with older adults are familiar with their state reporting laws for elder mistreatment. Medical providers are among the only people an isolated older adult may have contact with outside of the home. Sadly, studies reveal many medical providers never ask patients about elder abuse and few report it [41, 42].

Nearly every jurisdiction in the United States mandates elder abuse reporting. However, there is wide variation in the nuances of these laws, including who is a mandated reporter, what must be reported, timelines to report, where to report, and penalties for failing to report [43, 44]. Therefore, it is important for professionals to be aware of legal requirements where they practice to ensure that legal duties are satisfied. The Adult Protective Services Reporting Laws, prepared by the American Bar Association, highlights mandatory reporting laws by jurisdiction. It is available at https://www.americanbar.org/content/dam/aba/administrative/law_aging/2020-elder-abuse-reporting-chart.pdf. Additional reporting information is available at https://mandatedreporter.com/elder-abuse/.It is also important to know if there are other categories of mandatory reporting in a practice jurisdiction, e.g., unattended deaths, use of firearms, domestic violence, and child abuse that may be present in an elder abuse situation. If so, mandated reporters must meet all reporting requirements. Exceptions in some states for reporting domestic violence may not extend to domestic violence when committed against older or vulnerable adults. It may be helpful to consult a hospital or practice legal advisor when such situations arise.

Failure to report by a mandated reporter may be sanctioned as a crime, a licensing violation, and/or a civil breach of duty. Nearly every state provides criminal and civil immunity for good faith reporting. Additionally, anonymous reporting of suspected abuse as defined by local law is typically authorized for those who are not mandatory reporters.

In general, the identity of the reporter is confidential. However, if a case is prosecuted, the defendant's right to a fair trial and the prosecutor's duty to provide discovery often mean the reporter's identity and content of their report will be disclosed to the defense and if there is a trial, to the judge and or jury [45].

Navigating the Medico-Legal Interface

Medical providers are critical to proving criminal physical abuse cases. While court obligations can be time consuming and laborious, most prosecutors try to work with the clinician's schedule and limit the time needed for consultation and testimony. In communities with a medical provider on the Multidisciplinary Team (MDT), they may review medical records, interpret and explain findings, and follow up with providers with questions, resources, and observations related to capacity. This process helps to narrow the issues the clinician may need to address in a prosecution.

For Criminal Justice Professionals

Role of the Prosecutor

Prosecutors play a unique role in the criminal justice system. Unlike an attorney who practices civil law and represents an identifiable client, the prosecutor represents the members of the community in which they serve [45]. While in the civil justice arena the client can begin, end, or agree to resolve a matter, the victim in a criminal case has no similar authority over the prosecutor. A civil attorney, with the client's consent, may seek a civil protective order against the perpetrator or pursue civil causes of actions seeking relief and damages. Causes of action may include assault and battery, divorce, and elder abuse. In contrast, a prosecutor decides if the perpetrator should be charged with a crime. Civil actions typically lead to monetary awards; criminal prosecutions typically lead to court supervision, jail or prison terms, and for a few crimes, death sentences. Civil and criminal actions can be pursued simultaneously.

Assessing Whether the Case Is Provable

As with any physical abuse or other criminal case, the prosecutor decides who and what is charged. When evaluating charges the prosecutor determines: (1) if the case can be charged and if so, (2) whether it should be charged. The first involves an objective review of the evidence for its convincing force; the second balances the equities of filing a case once sufficient evidence to prove the case has been identified.

In physical abuse cases, like other types of elder abuse matters, the prosecutor can be helpful to, and be helped by, participation on an MDT. The MDT process can engage the prosecutor in the case at an early stage and provide a forum to consult with critical partners, including medical providers, law enforcement, APS, social workers, civil attorneys, and advocates. In doing so (1) victim needs and safety are addressed, (2) the victim is offered consistent support, and (3) critical case information is promptly identified and obtained.

MDT members can be helpful to prosecutors in evaluating if the victim can participate in the case. For example, if needed, qualified experts may conduct medical and capacity assessments or arrange for those evaluations to determine if the victim is competent to testify and identify procedures or accommodations that may allow them to testify most effectively. Members may be able to interpret medical evidence and offer expert testimony to overcome assumptions that the victim is not credible or does not understand what happened and to explain the science about the impact of trauma on a victim with a cognitive condition. Additionally, medically-trained MDT members may be able to help the prosecutor better understand the relationship between dementia, trauma, and memory.

When evaluating the sufficiency of evidence, the prosecutor reviews information provided by law enforcement and APS, including observations, statements from victims/clients, suspects, and witnesses, and documentary evidence. The prosecutor also evaluates ~~the~~ documentation from pre-hospital, ED, hospital, and outpatient medical providers. Pre-hospital clinicians' observations of the crime scene, condition of the victim and perpetrator, and statements by the victim and perpetrator can paint a vivid picture of the situation and help rule out possible justifications offered by the abuser. Medical providers documentation of their observations of the victim's injuries and statements are key to describing conditions. Ideally, this documentation offers medical opinions about causation and severity of injuries, opining about the likelihood of non-injury related causes of physical findings. Medical observations and documentation can make a case provable even if the victim is unavailable to participate in the prosecution. Documentation in the form of photographs, body charts, and physician and nurse notes, is especially valuable and persuasive in court.

While the nomenclature and elements of crimes vary across the country, states commonly have statutes relating to assault, elder or vulnerable adult abuse, domestic or family violence, and increasingly, strangulation. In analyzing whether a crime is prosecutable, prosecutors evaluate likely defenses that the alleged perpetrator may claim and the evidence that supports or refutes them. In physical abuse cases, the most common defenses are self-defense, denial that the events occurred, and claims that the acts were consensual.

When a claim of "self-defense" is offered the alleged perpetrator may assert that the victim came at them aggressively or attacked them first, and in response, they acted to defend themselves. Prosecutors, analyzing self -defense claims will consider location and nature of injuries, respective sizes and strengths of the parties, power dynamic between the parties, prior history of physical abuse, use of a weapon (including less obvious weapons, such as walkers, canes, wheelchairs, etc.).

If the alleged victim or perpetrator has dementia, it is important to know if they have previously exhibited aggressive or combative behavior or resistance to care and the functional effects of dementia on the individual.

Defense claims that the event never happened can take several forms. The perpetrator may claim the victim misunderstood or imagined what was occurring because of their cognitive impairment or medical condition. Consideration should be given to the time and setting in which the incident occurred (e.g in a dark room in the middle of the night when the older adult had just awakened vs. in a well-lit kitchen in the middle of the morning after breakfast); what preceded the incident (including potential acute triggers); any previous similar incidents; and what the alleged victim did and said while reacting to the situation.

Perpetrators may also argue that victim injuries were caused by something other than abuse, such as conditions resulting from thinning sun-exposed skin, bleeding caused by medications such as anticoagulants, bleeding from underlying medical conditions, or an accidental fall. The clinical assessment by medical professionals described above is essential to evaluating this defense. Careful, comprehensive consideration of all medications, comorbidities, location of injuries, such as areas not typically exposed to sun, their appearance, presence of swelling or pain, and the condition of skin in areas with apparent injuries, photographs, and laboratory testing is essential to assess the likelihood that findings have an etiology other than abuse.

Considerations Regarding the Role of the Victim in the Criminal Justice Process

It is commonly assumed that the victim must testify in a physical abuse case in order for it to be provable. While it may be easier to prove a case in which the victim testifies to their victimization, it is not always necessary.

Some victims desire prosecution and are willing to participate in the criminal justice process. More commonly, victims want the abuse to end and the abuser to receive help, but do not want to be involved a criminal prosecution. Most perpetrators of physical abuse are people the victim knows, loves, and/or trusts. The abuser may be the only significant person in the victim's life, and losing this relationship may lead to loneliness, isolation, and placement in a skilled nursing facility. Further, some victims feel pressure from family members or fear retaliation or further abuse if they participate in the criminal case. Some may have had negative experiences if they sought help decades earlier. Others are unaware of resources to help them live in safety and without violence.

The prosecutor must consider if the case can proceed without the victim's testimony. Even ~~if~~ when initially willing to testify, an older adult may change their mind, develop significant cognitive impairment, suffer a catastrophic health crisis, or die. If the victim's testimony is critical to proving the crime, absent the victim's participation, the case may not be provable.

Gaining a victim's trust of the criminal process starts with their first contact with responders. Are they treated with respect, and are their opinions, concerns, and goals acknowledged? Are they promptly offered safety alternatives to returning home to the abuser? Building trust continues when law enforcement, medical providers, prosecutors, and others who interact with the victim express empathy, listen and document victim concerns and wishes, and consistently focus on victim's safety and well-being, and with victim's consent, connect to a victim advocate who can provide support throughout the criminal case. The advocate can also help the victim apply for victim of crime benefits, accompany them to court and meetings with law enforcement and prosecutors, update court dates, and arrange ~~for~~ transportation to court.

Prosecutors who identify victim concerns and wishes, clarify the goals of prosecution, and seek common ground may increase a victim's willingness to participate in the case. Many victims feel the abuse would end if the abuser received treatment for substance use, mental health disorders, or other conditions. They will often acknowledge prior unsuccessful efforts to have the perpetrator enter treatment. When a prosecutor communicates that the likely case outcome aligns with the victim's desires that the perpetrator receives treatment or other help, the same victims are more willing to participate in a prosecution.

Considerations in Cases in Which the Victim Has Cognitive Impairment

While many who experience physical abuse in later life are independent and healthy, some are not. Evaluating an abuse case in which the victim has a cognitive impairment, should include the same comprehensive review of the sufficiency of the evidence as when there is no concern for the victim's cognitive ability. In addition, it is critical to consider whether their cognitive state will affect their ability to testify, if needed, and the prosecutor's case theory and charging decision.

A diagnosis of dementia does not necessarily preclude a victim or other witness from testifying. A determination of legal incompetence to testify requires a finding that their cognitive impairment renders them unable to distinguish between truth and fantasy and unable to communicate information. Many people with mild cognitive impairment and even moderate dementia are competent to testify.

Additionally, people with cognitive impairment may be credible reporters about abuse-related experiences. Memory for an emotional event, such as physical elder abuse, is a reserved cognitive ability often retained through early stages of Alzheimer's disease and related dementias [47]. Emotional memory is spared in many people with dementia, even with their loss of verbal and declarative memory [47]. Directly-experienced traumatic events are less likely to be forgotten over time than other types of memories [47]. Emotional arousal promotes long and short-term memory of story details. Flash-bulb memories of major events may be preserved better in older than younger persons, and can *at least* be partially spared in Alzheimer's disease [47]. Emotional memory is laid down in the brain differently from routine information. Memory loss in Alzheimer's Disease is associated with damage to the hippocampus that impairs encoding or storage of new memories. Emotional arousal and encoding of emotional memories activate the amygdala which may modulate memory storage elsewhere in the brain [47].

Considering Which Crimes to Charge in These Cases and Methods to Protect the Victim

In a physical abuse case such as the case study at the beginning of the chapter, the prosecutor may charge an array of assault, domestic or family violence, and elder abuse crimes. In order to protect the victim, when available, the court may issue protective orders that typically prohibit the perpetrator from having contact with the victim.

Many state and federal jurisdictions have enacted specific laws regarding strangulation which can be charged in addition to or in lieu of general assault, domestic/family violence, and elder abuse crimes. A map of strangulation legislation across the US is available at the https://www.strangulationtraininginstitute.com/resources/legislation-map/.

Considerations About Whether the Case Should Be Prosecuted

The previous section described how a prosecutor determines if a case can be charged. Assuming that a case can be proven beyond a reasonable doubt, the prosecutor must still decide if the case *should* be prosecuted. This question raises issues of justice and equity, including what is in the best interests of the victim, the perpetrator, and the community [47]. Cases involving violence or a history of abuse are frequently charged to protect the victim and the community, and to hold the perpetrators accountable.

In physical abuse cases considerations of what is just and equitable includes consideration of (1) the victim's desires and reasons; (2) the abuser's background and prior efforts to rehabilitate; (3) prior history of violence and intimate partner abuse; (4) available community alternatives to prosecution; (5) the fair and efficient use of prosecutorial resources; and (6) if community "interests can be appropriately vindicated by available civil, regulatory, administrative, or private remedies." [45]

Evaluating Alternatives to Prosecution and/or Incarceration

Not all physical abuse cases can or should be prosecuted and/or result in a jail or prison sentence. There is evolving interest in developing and using other ways to resolve cases. These alternatives seek to balance justice and safety with the victim's goals including providing the abuser with help to address underlying causes of their abusive actions and/or focus on repairing or improving the relationship between the victim and perpetrator [48].

In general, these alternatives can be grouped as: (1) court alternatives that do not result in a conviction; (2) alternatives to incarceration following a conviction; and (3) community-based alternatives that do not require the involvement of a prosecutor or a court. These alternatives are described in Table 2.2 below.

Not all of these options are available in every community. Some, such as referral to the Probate Court, are only appropriate when there is evidence that the defendant/perpetrator meets legal standards for a guardianship/conservatorship. Some perpetrators may be ineligible for certain options because of the nature of the offense

Table 2.2 Alternatives to prosecution and/or incarceration

Category	Examples
Court Alternatives That Do Not Result in a Criminal Conviction	Court referral to Pretrial Diversion Programs that impose conditions such as treatment and restitution which if successfully completed do not result in a conviction
	Court acceptance of Conditional or Deferred Pleas of Guilty and ordering conditions such as treatment and restitution but upon successful completion of conditions the court sets aside the conviction
	Referral of a case to Probate Court for appointment of a guardian/conservator for the defendant followed by dismissal of the criminal case (for defendants whose actions resulted from an organic medical condition such as dementia)
Post Conviction Alternatives that Do Not Result in Incarceration	Post-Conviction Diversion and Deferred Entry of Judgment in which following conviction a person is supervised by the court or a probation department with conditions such as treatment and restitution ordered. As long as person successfully completes terms imposed by court, person does not serve time in custody and guilty finding is set aside.
	Probation with conditions occurs post-conviction and after court imposes a sentence which includes conditions such as treatment and restitution and a suspended period of incarceration. If the person successfully completes the conditions of probation, they do not serve time in custody
Community Based Alternatives That Do Not Require the Involvement of a Court or Prosecutor	Restorative justice programs
	RISE (https://risecollaborative.org/the-need/)
	Alternative Dispute Resolution (e.g., mediation)

(e.g., involving violence or weapons), prior criminal history, etc. Finally, some cases may be so serious that only a criminal prosecution and conviction can achieve offender accountability and protection of the community.

Determining if prosecution should occur will be based on information about the perpetrator from family, friends, their attorney, as well as medical records, and previous APS investigations; court files concerning prior criminal conduct, and law enforcement investigative files.

Some perpetrators may have cognitive impairments, dementia, or an organic brain syndrome. These can affect impulse control and lead to behavior changes and can interact with ongoing mental health and substance use issues. In these infrequent situations responses focused on safety and quality of life for both parties are optimal. The prosecutor and other MDT members may have a role in developing community care solutions for the victim and perpetrator.

Case Discussion

Earlier in the chapter the case of Mary and James Johnson was introduced. Mary was transported to the hospital following a neighbor's call to police. There is information suggestive of a prior abuse history, and current report and observation of signs and symptoms consistent with domestic/family violence, physical elder abuse, and strangulation. The chapter concludes with how the medical and legal information presented will intersect in this case.

Following James' arrest, the case went to the prosecutor's office for a charging decision. The prosecutor noted that considerable evidence supports filing of charges. For example, Mary's report of prior abuse and her fear of James, her report of a history of domestic violence ~~as~~ corroborated by the neighbor, injuries consistent with Mary's account of what occurred and inconsistent with James' claim that Mary fell over the cat, and the locations of injuries are strong evidence that support ~~the~~ assault, physical abuse and family/domestic violence charges. Injuries to her left cheek and right eye corroborate her statement that she was struck in the face; the hoarseness, loss of consciousness, petechiae in her eyes, scalp and ear, as well as the bruises behind both ears strongly support that she was strangled. The documentation of the paramedics, ER and other medical providers, hospital social worker, and responding officers support the charges.

James will be afforded the opportunity to make a statement. Any information he may provide will be evaluated against other evidence and witnesses. Defenses will be weighed. Any indications that he may have medical or cognitive conditions which may have affected his ability to control his behavior will be considered.

If the community has an MDT, the prosecutor may consult with partners, including medical providers, law enforcement, Adult Protective Services, social workers and advocates, to address Mary's needs and safety. Medical providers may be asked to review and analyze medical records; any missing information will be identified and obtained, usually by law enforcement.

From earliest contact with the case, attention will be given to Mary's safety through protective orders to prohibit James from having any contact with her, connecting with Adult Protective Services, and linking her to community services for safety planning if she agrees. Additionally, advocates will contact Mary to assess her needs and concerns, explain the criminal process, determine if she needs any accommodations to meet with the prosecutor or provide testimony, update her on proceedings, and identify her desires regarding the case. Recognizing that criminal cases are stressful for victims like Mary, and may result in health changes, including premature death, the prosecutor will resist unnecessary delays in the process, and will likely memorialize her testimony early in the criminal process in case it is needed for later use at trial.

How would a case like Mary and James be resolved? The prosecutor would consider Mary's desires, needs and goals, along with information about James. Information from Mary related to case resolution would include: safety needs; does she wish to continue the relationship with James; is she dependent on him for her income, residence, daily activities, managing her finances and medical care; her expenses and losses from the victimization; her perceptions about why James may have abused her, e.g., medical, mental health, anger, or cognitive conditions, etc., and prior counselling or treatment James has had for these conditions. Information about James relevant to sentence would include criminal or mental health history, age, underlying medical or cognitive conditions, and willingness to accept responsibility for his actions.

It is likely that any sentence would include a no contact with Mary order, at least until completion of some portion of any court-imposed treatment, and a requirement that he make restitution for Mary's losses, including medical bills resulting from his conduct. If his conviction were for a felony or domestic violence offense, the court likely would be required to prohibit his possession or obtaining of firearms and ammunition under federal or state law, or both.

Key Points

- Though physical abuse is not the most common type of elder mistreatment, it can be particularly devastating for an older adult
- Though physical elder abuse may occur within a caregiving relationship, a typical victim often does not have substantial cognitive or functional impairment which differs from other mistreatment types such as neglect.

For Medical Professionals

- Because physical abuse may also occur in the context of domestic abuse/family violence, exploring medical history, asking about prior abuse, examining the patient alone and providing appropriate resources should be considered
- Radiographic imaging correlates for intentional injuries have been a critical element of child abuse detection but are only beginning to be explored as a potential tool in physical elder abuse

- Though forensic injury patterns highly specific for physical elder abuse have not yet been described in the literature, suggestive injury patterns exist that may help professionals assess injured older adults
- Strangulation may be involved in physical elder abuse, and injuries in the neck area or other suggestive features of the older adult should prompt consideration
- For many victims of physical elder abuse, the "false story" given for their injuries is a fall, which can occur commonly among older adults. It is, therefore, essential to consider whether physical findings exist after a reported fall that raise concern for abuse
- Taking photographs and documenting injuries and other physical findings are very helpful in proving physical abuse
- Considering an older adult's immediate safety and minimizing the risk of re-victimization are essential components of a professional assessment of physical elder abuse victims

For Criminal Justice Professionals

- Prosecutors evaluate cases in terms of provability (can case be charged) and equity (should the case be charged)
- Medical evidence and expert testimony are critical in determining if a physical abuse case can be proven
- Not all cases require that the victim testify
- Various alternatives are available to resolve a physical abuse case which may better align with a victim's wishes while protecting the community and holding offenders accountable
- Multidisciplinary teams are critical in building, evaluating, and resolving physical abuse cases and supporting victims.

For Social Work Professionals

- Psychosocial assessments are a valuable tool in being able to access for prior abuse and any type of successful treatment plans that were utilized in someone's past.
- Meet the older adult where they are in disengaging from the abuser.
- If the older adult wants to have any additional resources for care or assistance once discharge, provide appropriate referrals.
- Discharge planning to include a safety plan that can be implemented by the older adult or a trusted person in the older adult's life.
  - Discharge planning should include discharging to a safe location or one that is fully accessible to people who are deemed safe to the older adult

References

1. Acierno R, Hernandez MA, Amstadter AB, et al. Prevalence and correlates of emotional, physical, sexual, and financial abuse and potential neglect in the United States: the National Elder Mistreatment Study. Am J Public Health. 2010;100(2):292–7. (Research Support, N.I.H., Extramural Research Support, U.S. Gov't, Non-P.H.S.) (In eng). https://doi.org/10.2105/AJPH.2009.163089.
2. Lachs MS, Pillemer K. Elder abuse. Lancet. 2004;364(9441):1263–72. (In eng). https://doi.org/10.1016/S0140-6736(04)17144-4.
3. National Research Council. Elder mistreatment: abuse, neglect and exploitation in an aging America. Washington, DC: The National Academies Press; 2003.
4. Lifespan of Greater Rochester I, Weill Cornell Medical College, New York City Department for the Aging. Under the Radar: New York State Elder Abuse Prevalence Study. http://www.ocfs.state.ny.us/main/reports/Under%20the%20Radar%2005%2012%2011%20final%20report.pdf.
5. National center for Elder Abuse. What is elder abuse? Defining abuse. https://ncea.acl.gov/elder-abuse#gsc.tab=0.
6. Vandeweerd C, Paveza GJ. Verbal mistreatment in older adults: a look at persons with Alzheimer's disease and their caregivers in the state of Florida. J Elder Abuse Negl. 2005;17(4):11–30. (In eng). https://www.ncbi.nlm.nih.gov/pubmed/17050490.
7. Cooney C, Howard R, Lawlor B. Abuse of vulnerable people with dementia by their carers: can we identify those most at risk? Int J Geriatr Psychiatry. 2006;21(6):564–71. (In eng). https://doi.org/10.1002/gps.1525.
8. Amstadter AB, Zajac K, Strachan M, Hernandez MA, Kilpatrick DG, Acierno R. Prevalence and correlates of elder mistreatment in South Carolina: the South Carolina elder mistreatment study. J Interpers Violence. 2011;26(15):2947–72. (Research Support, N.I.H., Extramural) (In eng). https://doi.org/10.1177/0886260510390959.
9. Jackson SL, Hafemeister TL. Risk factors associated with elder abuse: the importance of differentiating by type of elder maltreatment. Violence Vict. 2011;26(6):738–57. (In eng). https://doi.org/10.1891/0886-6708.26.6.738.
10. Laumann EO, Leitsch SA, Waite LJ. Elder mistreatment in the United States: prevalence estimates from a nationally representative study. J Gerontol B Psychol Sci Soc Sci. 2008;63(4):S248–54. (Comparative Study Research Support, N.I.H., Extramural) (In eng) https://www.ncbi.nlm.nih.gov/pubmed/18689774.
11. Gottesman E, Elman A, Rosen T. Elder mistreatment: emergency department recognition and management. Clin Geriatr Med. 2023;39(4):553–73.
12. Lachs MS, Fulmer T. Recognizing elder abuse and neglect. Clin Geriatr Med. 1993;9(3):665–81. (In eng).
13. Ziminski CE, Wiglesworth A, Austin R, Phillips LR, Mosqueda L. Injury patterns and causal mechanisms of bruising in physical elder abuse. J Forensic Nurs. 2013;9(2):84–91; quiz E1-2. (In eng). https://doi.org/10.1097/JFN.0b013e31827d51d0.
14. Wiglesworth A, Austin R, Corona M, et al. Bruising as a marker of physical elder abuse. J Am Geriatr Soc. 2009;57(7):1191–6. (In eng). https://doi.org/10.1111/j.1532-5415.2009.02330.x.
15. Stevens TB, Richmond NL, Pereira GF, Shenvi CL, Platts-Mills TF. Prevalence of nonmedical problems among older adults presenting to the emergency department. Acad Emerg Med. 2014;21(6):651–8. https://doi.org/10.1111/acem.12395.
16. Elman A, Baek D, Gottesman E, et al. Unmet needs and social challenges for older adults during and after the COVID-19 pandemic: an opportunity to improve care. J Geriatr Emerg Med. 2021;2(11). https://doi.org/10.17294/2694-4715.1004.
17. Elman A, Rosselli S, Burnes D, et al. Developing the emergency department elder mistreatment assessment tool for social workers using a modified Delphi technique. Health Soc Work 2020 (In eng). https://doi.org/10.1093/hsw/hlz040.

18. Murphy K, Waa S, Jaffer H, Sauter A, Chan A. A literature review of findings in physical elder abuse. Can Assoc Radiol J. 2013;64(1):10–4. (In eng). https://doi.org/10.1016/j.carj.2012.12.001.
19. Collins KA. Elder maltreatment: a review. Arch Pathol Lab Med. 2006;130(9):1290–6. (In eng). https://doi.org/10.1043/1543-2165(2006)130[1290:EMAR]2.0.CO;2.
20. Collins KA, Presnell SE. Elder neglect and the pathophysiology of aging. Am J Forensic Med Pathol. 2007;28(2):157–62. (In eng). https://doi.org/10.1097/PAF.0b013e31805c93eb.
21. Collins KA, Sellars K. Vertebral artery laceration mimicking elder abuse. Am J Forensic Med Pathol. 2005;26(2):150–4.
22. Rosenblatt DE, Cho KH, Durance PW. Reporting mistreatment of older adults: the role of physicians. J Am Geriatr Soc. 1996;44(1):65–70. (In eng). https://www.ncbi.nlm.nih.gov/pubmed/8537593.
23. Gibbs LM. Understanding the medical markers of elder abuse and neglect: physical examination findings. Clin Geriatr Med. 2014;30(4):687–712. https://doi.org/10.1016/j.cger.2014.08.002.
24. Palmer M, Brodell RT, Mostow EN. Elder abuse: dermatologic clues and critical solutions. J Am Acad Dermatol. 2013;68(2):e37–42. (In eng). https://doi.org/10.1016/j.jaad.2011.03.016.
25. Chang ALS, Wong JW, Endo JO, Norman RA. Geriatric dermatology: part II. Risk factors and cutaneous signs of elder mistreatment for the dermatologist. J Am Acad Dermatol. 2013;68(4):533 e1–533 e10. https://doi.org/10.1016/j.jaad.2013.01.001.
26. Rosen T, Bloemen EM, LoFaso VM, Clark S, Flomenbaum NE, Lachs MS. Emergency department presentations for injuries in older adults independently known to be victims of elder abuse. J Emerg Med. 2016;50(3):518–26. https://doi.org/10.1016/j.jemermed.2015.10.037.
27. Rosen T, Clark S, Bloemen EM, et al. Geriatric assault victims treated at U.S. trauma centers: five-year analysis of the national trauma data bank. Injury. 2016;47(12):2671–8. https://doi.org/10.1016/j.injury.2016.09.001.
28. Rosen T, LoFaso VM, Bloemen EM, et al. Identifying injury patterns associated with physical elder abuse: analysis of legally adjudicated cases. Ann Emerg Med. 2020. (In eng). https://doi.org/10.1016/j.annemergmed.2020.03.020.
29. Stapczynski JS, Dietrich A. Strangulation injuries. Emerg Med Rep. 2010;31(17):193–203.
30. Faugno D, Waszak D, Strack GB, Brooks MA, Gwinn CG. Strangulation forensic examination: best practice for health care providers. Adv Emerg Nurs J. 2013;35(4):314–27.
31. De Boos J. Review article: non-fatal strangulation: hidden injuries, hidden risks. Emerg Med Australas. 2019;31(3):302–8. (In eng). https://doi.org/10.1111/1742-6723.13243.
32. Suffla S, Seedat M. The epidemiology of homicidal strangulation in the City of Johannesburg, South Africa. J Forensic Leg Med. 2016;37:97–107.
33. Rosen T, Bloemen EM, Harpe J, et al. Radiologists' training, experience, and attitudes about elder abuse detection. AJR Am J Roentgenol. 2016;207(6):1210–4. https://doi.org/10.2214/AJR.16.16078.
34. Wong NZ, Rosen T, Sanchez AM, et al. Imaging findings in elder abuse: a role for radiologists in detection. Can Assoc Radiol J. 2017;68(1):16–20. https://doi.org/10.1016/j.carj.2016.06.001.
35. Kempe CH, Silverman FN, Steele BF, Droegemueller W, Silver HK. The battered-child syndrome. JAMA. 1962;181:17–24. https://www.ncbi.nlm.nih.gov/pubmed/14455086.
36. Kleinman PK. Diagnostic imaging in infant abuse. AJR Am J Roentgenol. 1990;155(4):703–12. https://doi.org/10.2214/ajr.155.4.2119097.
37. Nimkin K, Kleinman PK. Imaging of child abuse. Pediatr Clin N Am. 1997;44(3):615–35. https://www.ncbi.nlm.nih.gov/pubmed/9168871.
38. LoFaso VM, Rosen T. Medical and laboratory indicators of elder abuse and neglect. Clin Geriatr Med. 2014;30(4):713–28. https://doi.org/10.1016/j.cger.2014.08.003.
39. Coulourides Kogan A, Rosen T, Homeier D, Chennapan K, Mosqueda L. Paper abstract-developing a tool to improve documentation of physical findings in injured older adults by health care providers: insights from experts in multiple disciplines. J Am Geriatr Soc. 2017;65:S1–S289.

40. Bloemen EM, Rosen T, Cline Schiroo JA, et al. Photographing injuries in the acute care setting: development and evaluation of a standardized protocol for research, forensics, and clinical practice. Acad Emerg Med. 2016;23(5):653–9. https://doi.org/10.1111/acem.12955.
41. Cooper C, Livingston G. Mental health/psychiatric issues in elder abuse and neglect. Clin Geriatr Med. 2014;30(4):839–50. (In eng). https://doi.org/10.1016/j.cger.2014.08.011.
42. Mosqueda L, Dong X. Elder abuse and self-neglect: "I don't care anything about going to the doctor, to be honest…". JAMA. 2011;306(5):532–40. (In eng). https://doi.org/10.1001/jama.2011.1085.
43. Thomas R, Reeves M. Mandatory reporting laws. StatPearls. Treasure Island (FL): StatPearls Publishing Copyright © 2024, StatPearls Publishing LLC.; 2024.
44. National Center on Elder Abuse. Mandated reporting of abuse of older adults and adults with disabilities. https://pfs2.acl.gov/strapib/assets/NCEA_NAPSA_Mandated_Report_Brief_915876f3dd.pdf.
45. *Brady v Maryland* (1963) 373 US 83, 83 S Ct 1194, 10 L Ed 2d 215; *U.S. v Bagley* (1985) 473 US 667, 676, 105 S Ct 3375, 87 L Ed 2d 481).
46. Berger v. United States (1935) 295 US 78; American Bar Association, Standards Related to the Prosecution Function, 3–1.2; ABA Criminal Justice Standards for the Prosecution Function (2017) Standard 3–1.3. available at https://www.americanbar.org/groups/criminal_justice/standards/ProsecutionFunctionFourthEdition/.
47. American Bar Association, Criminal Justice Standards for the Prosecution Function 2017, Standard 4.4 Discretion in Filing, Declining, Maintaining and Dismissing Criminal Charges. https://www.americanbar.org/groups/criminal_justice/standards/ProsecutionFunctionFourthEdition/.
48. Jackson SL, Heisler C, Urban K. A narrative review of US elder abuse perpetrator research and its implications for developing alternative perpetrator interventions for use by prosecutors. Aggress Violent Behav. 2024;76:101921.
49. Gascho D, Heimer J, et al. Forensic Imaging 22; Sept 2022.

Suggested Reading

Safarik ME, Jarvis JP, Nussbaum KE. Sexual homicide of elderly females: linking offender characteristics to victim and crime scene attributes. J Interpers Viol. 2002;17(5):500–25.
Wiglesworth A, Mosqueda L. People with dementia as witnesses to emotional events. Washington, DC: National Institute of Justice; 2011.

Chapter 3
Financial Exploitation

Mark Lachs, Kathy Van Olst, and Karen Webber Skuse

Introduction

A computer search for the terms elder abuse or elder mistreatment yields photographs and descriptions of physical injuries or of an abuser attacking an older person. That is what most people think when they hear the terms. Many epidemiological studies, however, suggest that financial exploitation is the most common form of elder abuse. There is a rising number of reported cases but a New York State Elder Abuse Prevalence Study, funded by NYS Office of Child and Family Services notes that the number reported is only the tip of the iceberg. (They estimate that for every case reported, there are 44 cases not reported, and that elder financial mistreatment affects 42 out of 1000 older New Yorkers") [1]. And, in the opinion of some experts, financial exploitation is the gateway to other forms of elder abuse. Although elder abuse is often considered primarily the concern of the medical team, a multidisciplinary perspective—medical, financial, and legal—is needed to uncover areas of financial exploitation that may go undiscovered and thus unresolved. Multidisciplinary teams (MDTs) are essential in helping to provide and bridge information. Working together, professionals can work quickly to end abuse.

M. Lachs (✉)
Division of Geriatrics and Palliative Medicine, Weill Cornell Medicine, New York, NY, USA
e-mail: mslachs@med.cornell.edu

K. Van Olst
District Attorney's Office, Seattle, WA, USA

K. W. Skuse
Founder, Fraudfindr, Rochester, NY, USA
e-mail: kwebber@bonadio.com

V. LoFaso, L. Rachmuth (eds.), *Elder Abuse and Neglect*,
https://doi.org/10.1007/978-3-031-97784-8_3

Case Presentation

The case of Michael R. was referred to the District Attorney's office for possible criminal charges following a law enforcement investigation of possible financial exploitation of an older adult by a caregiver.

Michael R. is a 95-year-old man who was born in Greece and immigrated to the United States in his early twenties. His wife, Maria R., died 4 years ago after 60 years of marriage. Their three adult children were in regular contact with both of their parents until Maria's death The entire family has strong ties to the local Greek Orthodox Church. Michael R. and his family also have a vacation home in California where he spends much of the winter. Michael R.'s children describe their father as frugal and financially conservative.

After his wife's death, Michael R. continued to live in the family home and to travel to California with his caregiver. The caregiver, who lives with Michael R., is a 45-year-old woman, an unlicensed home care assistant with no medical training, hired by the family from an internet site. She has three adult children. She originally helped care for Maria R. and assist Michael R. after her death as his needs increased. Prior to Maria's death, her primary care physician reported the caregiver to Adult Protective Services (APS) and Michael's children because of concerns about neglect and over-medication. Maria was moved to a nursing home shortly before her death. Michael R. insisted that the caregiver remain employed by him despite the objections of Maria's physician and his children. Michael R.'s decision to retain the caregiver caused considerable strain within the family and that strain reduced his contact with his children.

Michael R. had a stroke about 10 years ago that left him blind in his left eye. He had spinal and neck surgeries approximately 6 years ago, now uses a wheelchair and is hard of hearing. He had an abdominal aneurysm 4 years ago and was diagnosed with prostate cancer 2 years ago. Because of his spinal and prostate cancer issues, Michael R. uses a catheter full-time. For the past 8 years Michael has been prescribed medications for depression, blood pressure, leg cramping, pain, and sleep apnea, as well as muscle relaxants and blood thinners.

Michael R.'s children noticed that after the death of their mother, their father seemed to decline cognitively, to be depressed, and to increasingly rely on the in-home caregiver to cope with daily life. When a Mini Mental Status Exam was given to Michael R. by his physician a few years ago, he scored 20 out of 30, indicating memory loss or cognitive impairment. Michael R. regularly attends his scheduled medical appointments accompanied by his caregiver. Due to Michael R.'s cognitive decline, the caregiver provided his recent physical history. During appointments Michael nodded in agreement and only on occasion participated by answering direct questions.

While in California with his caregiver, Michael R. elected to have catheter repositioning surgery. At a post-operation visit 2 weeks after the surgery, the urologist found that the catheter had been dislodged and that his abdominal wall was infected. Michael R. was admitted to the hospital for two-and-a-half weeks to heal the infection. During his hospitalization, Michael R. developed delirium and that resulted in further cognitive decline. Hospital staff, concerned about his condition, called his son, a physician who holds his durable power of attorney. The caregiver had not notified any of his children of the surgery or hospitalization. Michael R'. children took over directing his care and returned him to the family home once he was well enough to travel.

Michael R. is currently continuing follow up treatment for his surgical complications. He is accompanied to medical visits by his son. At the present time, Michael is unable to accomplish most of the activities of daily living on his own and is unable to provide accurate medical history.

Financial History

Michael R., a strong-willed man who values his independence, lived independently with his wife until her death 4 years ago. He successfully ran his own business for many years and added to his wealth by investing in real estate.

After the loss of his wife, Michael R. became increasingly reliant on the caregiver for nearly all his daily activities including his finances. Three years ago, Michael R. and his caregiver opened a joint checking account with debit card and credit card access to allow the caregiver to buy Michael R.'s groceries, obtain his medications and pay his bills. Michael R. instructed the bank that this was the only account the caregiver could access. When Michael R.'s long-time accountant learned of the joint account, he met with Michael and the caregiver to confirm with both that this account was to be used for Michael's needs only and not for the caregiver's personal use. Both Michael and the caregiver agreed.

After the opening of the joint account, the bank manager noted that only the caregiver or her adult children came to the bank to access the account. When the family became aware of Michael R.'s hospitalization in California and re-assumed care of him, they discovered that the caregiver had the title to a car that was recently purchased by Michael in California. They also learned that there were extensive records of retail store purchases made during her employment using Michael R.'s money and that she was in possession of checkbooks for all his bank accounts. Based on the information the family gathered from the bank records, Michael R.'s children alerted local law enforcement of her actions and their concerns.

As part of the police investigation, a forensic accountant reviewed all of Michael R.'s bank records during the 4 years he employed the caregiver. The accountant and police confirmed with Michael R. and his children that he did not own a computer and that he did not know how to operate a computer to conduct online banking. Given that information, the accountant was able to identify at least 29 online transfers totaling $209,000.00 made by the caregiver from bank accounts belonging to Michael R. that the caregiver was not authorized to access. The caregiver deposited those transfers into the joint checking account and then spent it on items for her own benefit. The accountant also was able to determine that over the past 3 years, the caregiver spent over $322,000.00 of Michael R.'s money solely through online retail purchases for herself and her children. In addition, the accountant identified 123 checks written by the caregiver to her own adult children from Michael R.'s accounts without his knowledge. When he was questioned about the caregiver's banking and shopping, he was unaware of any of the questionable transactions.

Financial Exploitation Overview

One in five older adults has been the victim of financial abuse [2]. Older adults lose approximately $36 billion a year; the average individual loss is $120,300 [3]. More than one type of abuse can occur concurrently. The World Health Organization (WHO) estimates that 15.7% of people over 60 years of age and living in the community suffer some form of abuse: psychological 11.6%, financial 6.8%, neglect 4.2%, physical 2.5%, and sexual 1%.

In this Chapter, financial exploitation of an elder is defined as someone taking money or property from an older person without his or her knowledge, understanding, or consent [4]. Financial exploitation based on undue influence will be discussed in a later chapter.

Detecting elder financial exploitation can be challenging. When an older adult presents to a health care facility or professional there may be no obvious signs of abuse, and it may not be immediately evident that the elder is a victim of financial exploitation. Financial abuse is often discovered only through private conversations with the older adult or by observations by family, friends, or healthcare professionals about changes in the older adult's habits or behaviors or concerns about people newly or increasingly in control of the adult. Clues to the clinician about financial abuse might include medication non-adherence (if the older adult can no longer afford their medications), housing insecurity, weight loss, social isolation and depression.

The prevalence of dementia rises dramatically with age; dementia is now an epidemic in aging societies. At age 65 approximately 4% of tested individuals qualify for the diagnosis of either mild cognitive impairment or the formal diagnosis of dementia; at age 85 the prevalence rises to over 40%. Alzheimer's disease is regarded as the most common cause of dementia [5]. No matter what the cause of dementia, it typically affects several domains of cognition, including memory loss, calculational ability, inductive and deductive reasoning, and judgment. Each of these losses can impact financial decision making and increase vulnerability to financial exploitation. Financial exploitation may be an early manifestation of a dementing illness since declines in cognition typically precede impairments in activities of daily living (ADLS) and instrumental activities of daily living (IADLS) [1]. In some cases, financial exploitation may be the first, and for a time the only, manifestation of a dementing illness; extensive neuropsychological testing and radiological imaging reveal no abnormalities. Other typical stigmata of dementia eventually appear: short-term memory loss, gait changes, and word-finding difficulties.

In addition to dementing illness normal physiological changes of aging may increase the risk of financial exploitation [1]. The process, commonly referred to as Age Associated Financial Vulnerability, (AAFV) can be seen not only in patients/clients with a diagnosable dementing illness, but also in those who test normally after an extensive neurological evaluation but demonstrate loss of financial ability.

Many other factors than dementia, often in combination with each other and dementia, increase the risk of financial vulnerability: depression, social isolation and loneliness, and sensory or physical impairments. The patient, for example, may not be able to see well enough to read financial documents, may not be able to hear instructions, and may not be able to write clearly.

In general, older patients or clients who display changes in financial decision-making abilities that place them at risk for declining quality of life, should have medical and psychological evaluations. Physicians addressing cases such as Michael R.'s, should perform a complete medical evaluation to determine if patients merit a formal diagnosis of dementia, and if they do, to make sure that there are no reversible causes such as hypothyroidism, vitamin B12 deficiency, infection, or medication side effect. Often patients with dementia lack insight into their deficits (anosognosia) and refuse medical evaluation. In such cases, it will be important for the physician to collaborate with the patient, family, or healthcare proxy to ensure that they provide appropriate care and treatment.

Recognizing the Common Characteristics of the Perpetrator

More than 70 years ago, social researcher Donald Cressey conducted a survey of inmates who had been convicted of embezzlement to determine if there were any common characteristics among perpetrators that might indicate propensity to commit fraud. A theory called the Fraud Triangle was developed from his research. According to the Fraud Triangle Theory, three factors must be present for fraud to occur: opportunity (a person must be in a position of trust with very little oversight), pressure (from a "non-shareable personal problem" that a perpetrator would rather steal money to solve than seek help for), and rationalization (some reason a perpetrator finds to justify the theft). While the Fraud Triangle Theory was developed based on organizational crime, it applies to perpetrators of financial exploitation from a known person as well.

In this case, Michael R. relied heavily on the caregiver, slowly turning over to her all responsibilities for his care, including managing his finances. With her name on one of his accounts, the caregiver had an opportunity to help herself to his financial resources.

The caregiver created an unsustainable standard of living for herself with funds from Michael R. The pressure to keep up this lifestyle, as well as greed, may have motivated her to keep stealing from his accounts.

The caregiver could have made up any number of reasons to justify her crime when it first began—perhaps she felt entitled to it as a companion and possible status as a romantic partner; perhaps she felt she wasn't compensated enough for all the time she was spending with him; perhaps she thought she was just borrowing it at first, or that Michael R. would have wanted her to have it in the end.

When financial exploitation is committed by family members, as often happens [6], the Fraud Triangle factors may appear to be different. Trust may be automatic in a parent-child or grandparent-grandchild situation, and access to assets creates opportunity. Pressure to take a relative's money often comes from the potential perpetrator's addiction, failure-to-launch, or significant expenses they're unable to keep up with. When the potential perpetrator can somehow justify the taking of funds—"I would inherit this anyway", or "I provide so much unpaid work caregiving that I should be compensated"—the situation is ripe is for fraud.

A second theory, the Fraud Diamond, developed in 2000, expanded the fraud triangle to include capability as a fourth factor or tipping point necessary for the commitment of fraud [7] The theory posits that while opportunity, pressure, and rationalization are all necessary for financial exploitation, a prospective perpetrator must have certain characteristics to carry out fraud. Those characteristics include:

- knowledge of the system: how a potential victim's finances are managed
- knowledge of gaps in protective controls: that there is a lack of oversight of the management of the potential victim's finances by the victim or any other party
- knowledge that they are in a unique position to exploit the situation
- confidence that they can accomplish the theft and influence accomplices
- ability to lie to authority (victim, family, professionals, intervening agencies) if questioned

Case Discussion

In this case, Michael R.'s caregiver had access to certain accounts, knew how to access them, and knew also that neither Michael R. nor his geographically distanced children ever monitored activity. When questioned about the joint account by Michael R.'s accountant, she convincingly lied about the pretenses under which it was opened—a perfect example of the Fraud Diamond theory.

Earlier research on perpetrators in elder abuse cases centered on what became known as the caregiver stress theory, which suggests that caregivers who became overwhelmed by their responsibilities were at increased risk of abusing the older adult in their care [7]. Review of literature published in later years found that, in addition perpetrators of elder abuse of all types were more likely to be under age 60, white, unemployed, unmarried, and without children. Specific to financial exploitation, perpetrators frequently had problems with alcohol, gambling, and financial difficulties [8]. In Michael R.'s case, the common risk factors were the caregiver's age, race, and unmarried status.

Critically important to note is that perpetrators cannot be considered a homogenous group of simply bad actors. In most cases, perpetrators of abuse are made, not born. A 2016 study of 336 perpetrators in Illinois put perpetrators in four categories: [8].

- Caregivers—abusers who provide a positive emotional support and personal needs care for the victim.
- Dependent Caregivers—abusers who provide positive emotional support and personal needs care for the victim, and, most important, also rely on them financially, have difficulty keeping a job, and exhibit irresponsible behaviors. Interestingly, these abusers often have drinking problems.
- Temperamental—abusers who are not caregivers and who exhibit volatile behavior in their relationship with the victim, often including emotional conflict and bouts of temper.
- Dangerous—abusers who are not caregivers and who exhibit volatile behavior in their relationship with the victim, are emotionally draining for the victim, and frequently have trouble with the law.

Abusers who are caregivers, dependent or not, are more likely to commit emotional abuse. Those deemed Temperamental and Dangerous abusers are more likely to commit physical abuse. Dependent caregivers and Dangerous abusers are more likely to commit financial exploitation. (While Michael R.'s caregiver would not fit the classification of Dangerous as posed by DeLiema, she was certainly a Dependent Caregiver.

Frameworks like the Abuse Intervention Model help physicians understand risk factors in financial abuse.

Approaching a Financial Investigation

Setting Expectations: Information regarding the victim, the perpetrator, and the context of their relationship is usually gathered at the start of a case investigation. The questions posed and habits observed by the investigator need to establish expectations of the victim's normal behavior or expected activities.

Initial questions should focus on lifestyle—how does the victim spend his days? How does the victim spend his money? In Michael R.'s case, he was incredibly frugal despite his significant wealth. Monthly expenses outside of maintaining his homes were only $1790 per month, an amount more than covered by his income of about $10,000 per month.

If it becomes clear that another individual engages in managing the victim's finances to any degree, follow-up questions related to specific permissions given to that individual are helpful in assessing which transactions observed in the victim's financial records might or might not be reasonable or expected. Michael R.'s case was complex because he had given specific permission to the caregiver years ago to use his debit/credit card, use his car, and in some cases, pay for her personal medical expenses. And patients have the right to self-determination and to direct the use of their money. Even though investigators and Michael R's family may perceive the caregiver's spending as inappropriate, it was authorized by Michael R. prior to significant cognitive impairment and could not be held against the perpetrator during prosecution. The spending that he did not direct, the spending by the perpetrator outside of the permissions granted her, are what constituted financial exploitation.

Beyond questions, observations made about the victim's hygiene, the state of his or her home, or the presence of others living in the home can be important pieces of evidence in building a case of financial exploitation. Investigators visiting Michael R. noticed that none of his own children came to visit; instead, the caregiver's children were frequently in and out of the house, even removing food from the refrigerator so that there was not much left for Michael R. Worse, his once-impeccable home had fallen into a state of disrepair that did not reflect Michael R.'s apparent means.

All the questions, answers, and observations gathered at intake and as the case evolves provide the critical context to the story that the financial records will eventually illustrate as the investigation unfolds.

Collecting Financial Evidence

Financial records are necessary evidence in financial exploitation cases. These records might include checking, savings, digital forms of payment, brokerage, loan, credit card statements, tax returns, property records, any other evidence of financial transactions, and supporting records. Supporting records, in the context of banks, credit unions, digital banks/payment applications, and other depository institutions, usually mean:

- Account opening/change documents, sometimes called signature cards. These documents provide a sample of the victim's signature, indicate when the account was opened, and when another individual—the caregiver in Michael R.'s case—may have been added to the account as a joint owner, authorized user, or beneficiary. Account opening documents provided by the bank showed that Michael R.'s caregiver was a joint owner, which in many states allowed her ownership over some or all of the assets in the account. Generally, if she had been listed only as an authorized user, she would not have ownership, but she would have the authority to conduct transactions.
- Deposit slips and deposit items. When a deposit is made at a financial institution, a slip is filled out to indicate the amount deposited, whether it was cash or checks, and whether cash was provided during the transaction. Deposit items are copies of the checks that were deposited along with that slip. Deposit items are important for identifying other assets like accounts that were liquidated or may still

exist, reverse mortgage proceeds, proceeds from the sale of real property, insurance proceeds for policies that were canceled or liquidated, or proceeds from insurance claims of missing valuables. In Michael R.'s case, though the caregiver was a joint owner, none of the funds added to the account during the period were hers. All funds spent from the account were Michael R.s.

- Withdrawal slips are completed for withdrawals of cash or cashier's check from a teller at a financial institution. The slip indicates how much was withdrawn and who signed for it. Often, the individual making the withdrawal is required to sign the withdrawal slip. Most withdrawal slips do not indicate whether the funds were withdrawn as cash or a cashier's check, so requesting copies of all cashier's checks is recommended to determine where the certified funds were sent. In every instance in Michael R.'s case, the withdrawal slips were signed by the caregiver.
- Copies of canceled checks (front and back) are hugely important. Bank statements simply show that a check was cashed on a certain date for a certain amount. Generally, the statements show no details about to whom the check was made out, only the actual checks can do that. The front of the check provides evidence in the form of handwriting, payee instructions, signature, and memo details. The back of the check provides evidence in the form of what is called the endorsement—the signature or stamp of the payee, the bank where it was deposited, and in some cases, the exact account number where the funds were deposited. This information may help identify additional accounts owned by either the victim or the suspect for which records should be requested. Analysis of the copies of canceled checks provided by Michael R.'s bank showed that checks were written to the caregiver; endorsement details on the back of those checks indicated that the funds were deposited at a separate bank, leading investigators to the separate account the caregiver had set up to funnel Michael R.'s assets into her ownership.
- Transfer details/offsets are supplementary information that a financial institution maintains in its internal database which show the origin/destination account numbers & financial institutions for transfers between accounts. Transfer details are also necessary for a thorough investigation and were a critical piece of evidence in Michael R.'s case because transfers were another way that the caregiver moved money from Michael's accounts to her own.
- Power of Attorney documents on record, and non-depository accounts like mortgage and loan statements, digitally signed documents, and records are also helpful for painting a complete picture of the activity during the period of exploitation. This list is far from exhaustive.
- Considerations should be made when on-line banking is the mode of the financial transactions.

Banking and consumer privacy laws require the possible victim's consent for a third party—and investigator—to access the alleged victim's financial records. These laws make it difficult for concerned parties to investigate financial exploitation because older adults may not be capable of giving consent. Guardians, Conservators,

Power of Attorneys, Law Enforcement, and Adult Protective Services, however, have legal authority to obtain this information from financial institutions when fraud is suspected. In Michael R.'s case, financial records were obtained by law enforcement via subpoena. Those records contained bank statements that detailed the extent of the caregiver's activity over several years.

A good rule of thumb for requesting financial records from financial institutions is to ask for records, in writing, dating 6 months prior to the perpetrator's involvement, if that date is known, to the present time. If the perpetrator's approximate date of involvement is not known, the investigator could start by requesting the most recent 2 years and evaluate later whether additional records are needed. Requests should specifically indicate that the records to be produced include all accounts held individually or jointly by the alleged victim.

No matter how complex the older adult's assets are, information often winds up flowing through simple checking and savings accounts, which is frequently the perpetrator's original point of access. Investigators should be prepared: almost inevitably, investigators will find additional accounts, will find that pages and supporting records are missing and that further requests of more records are required. In Michael R.'s case, the caregiver was given access to a checking account, and evidence of the exploitation flowed from there.

Records Analysis: When the records requests are made of the financial institution and the documents are received, the analysis phase of the investigation begins. In the analysis phase, the investigator compares expectations gathered at intake to evidence contained in the financial records primarily using transactions performed during the period of investigation. In Michael R.'s case, a significant amount of time was spent by investigators performing transaction analysis, looking at transactions both individually and in aggregate to identify patterns and anomalies. Transaction analysis can be done manually or using software, often both. Patterns within the victim's accounts that should raise red flags for investigators include:

- Deviations from expectations
- Negative cash flow (withdrawals exceeding deposits)
- Decreasing monthly/annual deposits
- Increasing monthly/annual withdrawals
- Large, unknown withdrawals
- Transfers to/from other accounts unknown to the victim
- Frequent account changes (ex: new account numbers or new banks)
- Account ownership changes during period (ex: Power of Attorney added)
- Premature redemption of certificates of deposit, annuities, life insurance policies
- Inconsistent or suspicious handwriting or signatures on checks

Patterns within the perpetrator's accounts that should raise red flags for investigators include:

- Lack of regular wages (perhaps indicating no employment)
- Negative cash flow
- Overdraft fees

- Increasing monthly/annual deposits from victim funds
- No spending for household/grocery expenses (perhaps indicating these expenses are being covered by the victim)
- Spending above income level or previous patterns of spending
- Transfers to/from other accounts
- Similar purchases to those observed in Victim's accounts
- Similar handwriting or signatures to those observed in victim's accounts.
- Transactions indicative of pressure or motive (ex: casinos, liquor stores, inappropriate clothing)
- New digital spending/on-line purchases

Note that transaction data alone is not enough to determine financial exploitation—understanding the financial activity in the context of each specific case is critical for effective intervention. Whether the accounts being analyzed belong to the victim or the perpetrator, results of the analysis should clearly show a change in banking activity when alleged perpetrator became involved. In Michael R.'s case, debit card spending increased significantly after the caregiver was added to the account, and the locations where the card was being used did not align with what investigators knew about Michael's regular habits. In fact, once the defendant could use the bank account, the average spending for the household jumped from $1790 per month to $12,230 per month.

Use of Forensic Accountants or Financial Analysts

Most investigators in financial exploitation cases are social services and law enforcement workers, and their formative education was not in accounting, finance, asset tracing, business or property law. Because of this, records analysis is often a task left for experts like forensic accountants or financial analysts. In Michael R.'s case, the prosecutor's office had its own financial analyst on staff to develop the evidence used to charge the caregiver for her crime. Not many prosecutors' offices across the United States have such resources, so the work of financial analysis is outsourced to forensic accountants. Use of forensic accountants for financial exploitation cases is growing in popularity across the United States via various multidisciplinary structures [9, 10]. Forensic accountants and financial analysts can assist in all phases of the investigation: advising on which documents to collect, providing questions to ask in interviews, reviewing records, and even testifying in court as to their findings.

Use of Software: For investigators comfortable with or curious about doing their own transaction analysis, software may help. Common programs include:

- Spreadsheet tools like Excel® for inputting, sorting, and analyzing transactions
- Optical character recognition (OCR) tools convert transaction data from bank statements to a spreadsheet

- Data analysis tools that upload, read, and analyze financial transaction data for specific purposes

Specific to financial exploitation investigations, investigators should ensure that any method of analysis includes the ability to look at transactions individually and in aggregate to find patterns and anomalies.

Legal Considerations in Elder Financial Exploitation Cases

Elder financial exploitation is often a criminal matter. Historically, however, elder financial exploitation cases were considered family or civil court matters. Criminal cases, unlike family or civil ones, involve a governmental agency charging an individual (referred to as a defendant) with a crime, such as theft or financial fraud. If the defendant is found guilty of the crime, that individual often serves time in jail or prison, may have to complete certain requirements such as treatment or be on probation, and pay money which is referred to as restitution to the victim of the crime. Because society and law enforcement previously viewed the financial abuse of older adults as a financial dispute between two adults, it was thought of as civil matter to be handled in civil court.

Over the last few decades society has increasingly recognized that financial exploitation of older adults may constitute a crime and as such is appropriately overseen in the criminal justice system. Specifically, elder financial mistreatment involves a perpetrator targeting an older adult due to age or disability to obtain money or assets in violation of a trusted relationship with them or as a stranger [11]. Law enforcement and prosecutors view the perpetrator's actions in unlawfully taking, deceiving, or embezzling the assets of the older adult through the lens of state and federal criminal laws to determine whether to file criminal theft, fraud or exploitation charges against the perpetrator in criminal court.

Unlike most cases of financial exploitation where the perpetrator is known to the victim, scams are a bit different in that the perpetrator is often unknown to the victim. Scams will be discussed in the next section.

The filing of criminal charges in an elder exploitation case does not prevent civil attorneys from also pursuing remedies for the victim in court particularly in cases where the older victim may suffer cognitive decline impairing the ability to manage personal finances. Criminal theft charges may be filed against the perpetrator in criminal court and simultaneously, civil attorneys may file a civil conservatorship or guardianship, which gives a person partial or full decision-making authority over another person. Such a proceeding, in civil court, prevents the perpetrator from continued illegal access and control over the victim's assets. Even in cases where the victim suffers no cognitive issues, a victim of financial exploitation is often in need of a prosecutor in the criminal justice system to hold the perpetrator accountable for committing a crime and a civil legal attorney to assist them in repairing their credit, recovering stolen assets, and recovering for other damages that occurred because of the exploitation. It is increasingly common, therefore, for law enforcement and prosecutors working on criminal cases to work with civil attorneys on civil cases to address the past exploitation of the older adult and to prevent further victimization.

In Michael R.'s case, his children pursued both criminal and civil court action once they became aware of the caregiver's thefts and her undue influence over their father. In the criminal arena they reported their suspicions regarding the caregiver's financial exploitation of their father directly to police who obtained an immediate court order for records relating to Michael R.s financial accounts to investigate the allegations. Because of Michael R.'s apparent cognitive decline, which affected his ability to handle his finances and care for his own daily needs, his children took over management of his assets and health care as his powers of attorney. The power of attorney documents had been signed years earlier as part of Michael R.'s estate planning long before the onset of any cognitive impairment. Michael R.'s children also applied for a protection order in civil court to prevent the caregiver from contact with their father to stop any additional victimization.

Scams

Scams, also known as financial fraud is defined as acts that "intentionally and knowingly deceive the victim by misrepresenting, concealing, or omitting facts about promised goods, services, or other benefits and consequences that are nonexistent, unnecessary, never intended to be provided, or deliberately distorted for the purpose of monetary gain" [12].

Some of the most common scams perpetrated against older adults today are:

- The Grandparent scam: fraudsters call an older adult pretending to be a grandchild in trouble. They ask for money and request that the older adult doesn't tell the grandchild's parents.
- The Romance scam: fraudsters contact older adults online or via phone and begin building what feels like a romantic relationship. It isn't long after trust is established that they begin to ask for money. Pig butchering is one the many teams used to describe romance scams.
- Lottery and sweepstakes scams trick older adults into believing that they've won a sum of money, but first they must pay some of that money up front, such as for taxes.
- False investment schemes: fraudsters pitch an investment opportunity to older adults. Instead of using the money for building the business or buying the property they allege, the fraudster takes the money and uses it personally.
- Government imposter scams: fraudsters impersonate IRS, Medicare, or other official representatives and asking for personally identifiable information that can be used for identity theft.
- Charity scams were on the rise during the COVID-19 pandemic, as fraudsters sought donations for charities that didn't exist.

Other scams may involve fake products and services such as:

- Healthcare/Medicare/Health Insurance Fraud
- Counterfeit prescription drugs
- Funeral and cemetery scams
- Fraudulent anti-aging products
- Internet scams
- Telemarketing scams

Cryptocurrency scams are on the rise. The FBI's annual Elder Fraud Report revealed that older Americans lost over $3 billion in crypto fraud in 2022. Scams involving cryptocurrency are just like scams involving traditional currency:

- Investment schemes: promise substantial returns from assets that don't exist.
- Rug pull scam: investment scammers tout a new project, then disappear with funds after the older adult invests.
- Romance scams: instead of asking for cash, the scammer convinces victim to buy or give money in the form of cryptocurrency. Pig-butchering can be a form of a romance scam [13].
- Phishing scams: scammers send emails with malicious links to gather personal details, such as cryptocurrency wallet key information.
- Giveaway scams: come over the internet with links that lead to fraudulent site asking for verification to receive bitcoin which usually includes making payment to prove victim's account is legitimate.
- Ponzi scheme: a form of investment scam that pays older investors with proceeds from new ones. Ponzi schemes can be committed with traditional currency or cryptocurrency.
- Fake cryptocurrency exchanges: scammers lure investors in promises of great crypto gains when there no actual exchange exists

Cryptocurrency

Unlike cash, digital currency is actually traceable thanks to its existence on the blockchain. Because of this, it's marketed in some cases as safer than regular currency. However, like any other global currency, it fluctuates.

Fraud risks associated with digital currency:

- Like cash, it can be stolen through scams or unauthorized access.
- ICO, (Initial Currency Offering) is an IPO (Initial Public Offering) for a new currency. Asking for cash as part of a fake ICO is basically an investment scam.
- Phishing and Malware schemes: fraudsters create fake emails that look like your exchange or wallet and trick you out of your private keys, or access credentials, or lock your computer to compel you to turn them over

Locating Digital Assets

If you are assisting with an investigation and need assistance locating digital assets, secure the victim's digital devices and locate digital wallets. Analyzing email and browsing history may show purchase confirmations, bookmarks for online platforms, or conversations on Reddit or other forums that indicate current or former holdings. Consider interviewing friends and family for knowledge. If the victim held any cryptocurrency, law enforcement can subpoena exchanges for records of transactions stored on the blockchain. Blockchain analysis software can search for transactions and origin and destination account detail. IP addresses associated with those accounts may lead to the identity theft.

Under-Reporting of Financial Victimization in the Elderly

While it may seem obvious that reporting possible victimization is the critical first step in seeking justice for financial exploitation victims, reporting often fails to occur in these cases for many different reasons. A New York study in 2011 revealed that for every case of self-reported elder abuse, approximately 24 cases were not reported to any service provider in the elder services network [14] For cases of elder financial exploitation, only one out of 44 cases were ever reported to agencies serving elder abuse victims.

Victims of financial abuse often acknowledge hesitation to report the abuse. Some victims state that they fail to report the abuse because of an emotional dependence on a perpetrator, a fear of the loss of independence due to a loss of assets, a feeling of shame for falling victim to the perpetrator, and, if suffering from declining cognitive, a failure to recognize or believe that abuse is occurring. Particularly when elders may be suffering from loneliness and social isolation, victims may seek to maintain contact with perpetrators of financial exploitation because the perpetrators are often family members, caregivers, known associates such as pastors, powers of attorney, guardians, neighbors, investment advisors, and even strangers who have groomed the victim into believing that they will protect them.

Given the complex reasons why an older victim may fail to report this crime, detection and reporting of fraud often falls to individuals who are in contact with older adults and are knowledgeable about the signs and symptoms of the abuse. Many states designate these trusted individuals as mandatory and discretionary reporters of abuse. While the law in each state is different regarding who is tasked with being a reporter of elder abuse, individuals such as health care professionals, law enforcement, social workers, and, sometimes, bank employees are often identified as reporters. These individuals are most likely to be trained to talk with and to question the victim in a sensitive manner and in a trusted setting and to make observations regarding the victim and changes in the victim's life that suggest abuse has taken place. Victim lifestyle or behavioral changes are often designated as red flags or potential signs and symptoms of financial abuse. Red flags include estrangement from family and friends, a new controlling best friend, a caregiver or love interest who isolates and controls the elder, significant changes in spending patterns, non-payment of bills, missed medical appointments, and deterioration in self-care. While these red flags are only suggestive of abuse and do not prove that abuse has occurred, if they provide reasonable suspicion that abuse is occurring, state law often requires a report of abuse to be made to law enforcement or APS. Only after a report of abuse has been made to law enforcement or APS will specially trained investigators begin their evaluation of the abuse allegations.

In Michael R.'s case, the first report to law enforcement and APS came from his family after learning of Michael R.'s out-of-state hospitalization and of the caregiver's substantial use of Michael R.'s assets. While the treating physician at the out-of-state hospital did not report the caregiver for neglect, the physician called Michael R.'s family because of the severity of his condition and that call precipitated the family's intervention. At the time of the family's report of neglect and financial exploitation, the victim was unable to report because he was suffering from significant cognitive decline and was emotionally dependent on the perpetrator, his long-time caregiver. Michael R.'s family and law enforcement both reported allegations of neglect and financial abuse to APS.

Specialized Investigations Initiated by a Report of Elder Financial Exploitation

After a report of possible elder financial exploitation is received by law enforcement and Adult Protective Services (APS), both entities begin investigations. Additional agencies such as long-term care ombudsman and federal and state agencies may also be notified by law enforcement of the abuse allegations and open investigations. The two local agencies with primary investigative responsibilities in elder abuse cases, however, are typically APS and local or federal law enforcement. It is the duty of law enforcement and APS to investigate reports of suspected elder financial mistreatment to determine if there is validity to the allegations.

APS is a state program whose mission is directed primarily by state laws and regulations. In most states, APS is assigned to investigate reports of financial exploitation of vulnerable adults. APS investigations are not criminal investigations but rather administrative investigations that determine if the alleged facts support or fail to support allegations of wrongdoing. APS social workers interview the possible victims and witnesses and collect medical records and financial records in exploitation cases. If APS concludes that financial exploitation has occurred and is able to prove it by a preponderance of the evidence in an administrative hearing, then the perpetrator of the wrongdoing is entered into a state registry that disqualifies the offender from being licensed or employed to work with older and vulnerable adults. APS is also tasked with working with older and vulnerable adults to determine if they need services to meet their daily activities of life and if so, connecting them with appropriate resources.

Law enforcement, on the other hand, after receiving a report of elder financial exploitation, is tasked with investigating whether a crime occurred based on all available evidence. As part of the law enforcement investigation, police will contact the older adult to take an in-depth statement of what is alleged to have occurred. Police also will take witness statements from other individuals who may have relevant information such as bank personnel, family members, neighbors and long-term associates of the victim. Police will gather pertinent documents such as financial records and medical records in exploitation cases. Because law enforcement and APS often need similar information for their investigations, the agencies will share information as it is collected. Upon the conclusion of the police investigation, all the statements of witnesses and collected materials are forwarded to a prosecutor or District Attorney with a law enforcement recommendation for filing or not filing criminal charges.

In Michael R.'s case, after the report of financial exploitation by the family to law enforcement, the police undertook the primary investigation in the case. While APS opened an investigation into the allegations, APS decided to defer their administrative investigation until the law enforcement investigation was concluded.

Law enforcement interviewed Michael R. and found that while he was unaware of the facts underlying the allegations of elder financial mistreatment by the caregiver, he could provide background information that was helpful to the investigation. Based on the information provided in the initial family report and during Michael R.'s interview, law enforcement gathered additional evidence to assess the veracity of the financial mistreatment allegations such as witness statements from bank personnel, from Michael R.s long-time accountant, from his physician and from many members of his family. In addition, law enforcement obtained court orders to obtain bank and medical records during the period of the caregiver's employment. Based on the evidence law enforcement was able to collect, they forwarded their case to the prosecutor with a recommendation that theft charges be filed against the caregiver.

The Decision to File Charges and Prosecute Financial Abuse

Once a prosecutor receives a report of an elder financial exploitation investigation from law enforcement, the prosecutor must decide if a criminal case can and should be charged. The role of the prosecutor is to review all the materials gathered by police and APS and to undertake additional investigation if needed to determine if criminal charges can be filed against the alleged perpetrator. To file charges, the prosecutor must have witnesses available to present live testimony in court and relevant documents such as medical and financial records to convince a jury beyond a reasonable doubt that the perpetrator committed the charged crime.

The prosecutor's role also includes consideration of the equitable issues involved in charging a case. Unlike civil cases where the civil attorney files a case on behalf of a client, in criminal cases the prosecutor represents the government, and it is the prosecutor's responsibility to seek justice for the victim and for the community. While the prosecutor does not represent the victim, it is important for a prosecutor to consider the wishes of the older adult victim about whether to prosecute a case. Because elder financial cases involve adult victims who typically have control over their own assets and have the right to spend their money as they wish if they have financial capacity, prosecutors generally give greater deference to the victim's wishes in deciding whether to charge a financial exploitation case than in other types of elder abuse cases. Even in cases in which older adults have mild or moderate dementia and may not have capacity to make complex financial decisions, the victims may still have the capacity to understand and to express strong feelings about filing charges and the impacts of a criminal prosecution, particularly if the perpetrator is a family member.

In Michael R.'s case, because law enforcement recommended that the caregiver be charged with a crime, the prosecutor received the complete law enforcement investigation with all the medical and financial records to review. The severity of Michael's cognitive impairment made it necessary for the prosecutor to assess whether charges could be filed and proven without relying on his testimony at trial. Based on the prosecutor's review of all the witness testimony and the documentary evidence, the prosecutor concluded that criminal theft charges could be filed and proven against the caregiver. Before filing charges, the prosecutor talked with Michael R. about his wishes regarding prosecuting the caregiver given her long-term employment with him. Because he did not express any opinions for or against prosecuting the case, the prosecutor filed theft charges against the caregiver.

Need for Cooperation Among Healthcare, Financial, and Legal Professionals: A Multidisciplinary Response

The legal team will lead the prosecution, but the medical and financial professionals are needed to bring it to a successful conclusion.

Medical professionals are usually essential witnesses in elder financial abuse cases. Reports of suspected elder financial exploitation can involve situations in which family or friends question the appropriateness of decisions made by older adults regarding their spending decisions. If the elderly have the capacity to make informed decisions, those cases are not appropriate for criminal prosecution. Criminal prosecution in elder financial cases typically falls into two case types: (1) cases where the victim has capacity to make financial decisions and their assets are taken without their permission or without their knowledge; and (2) cases where victim's assets are taken and the victim is suffering from some level of cognitive impairment which impedes the ability to consent to the use or taking of their assets or to know that assets are being taken. Most, by far, of the elder financial exploitation reports to police involve older victims who have cognitive impairment. Medical evidence regarding the victim's cognitive functioning is, therefore, essential in proving the financial exploitation case and in defeating the usual defense in these cases—that the victim consented to the use of his or her assets.

Medical evidence in a financial exploitation case is critical in establishing the victim's physical and mental conditions during the time period of the exploitation so that juries can understand how the victim was vulnerable to the perpetrator's actions. Testimony of health care professionals about their interactions with victims, including documentation of office visits in medical records, provide a picture of changes in a victim's cognitive functioning over time. Types of documentation typically found in medical records, and relied upon in financial abuse cases, include information about signs and symptoms of cognitive impairment, statements by patients or family regarding cognitive functioning and behavioral concerns, and even statements by individuals accompanying the older patient that demonstrate attempts to inappropriately control the older adult's decision-making. As noted by a Canadian physician, family physicians are, by virtue of their frequent contact and trusting relationship with older adults, are uniquely positioned to identify and comprehensively document signs and symptoms suggestive of mistreatment [15].

Mental health professionals are essential in proving many elder financial mistreatment cases. Cognitive impairment and capacity experts can provide testimony regarding the victim's mental status during the exploitation, including such issues as whether the victim had the capacity to understand financial transactions, whether the victim's cognitive impairment would have been obvious to the perpetrator, and whether the victim was vulnerable to undue influence or deception by the perpetrator as a result of cognitive decline. The opinions of these experts typically are based on the victim's medical records and include their own cognitive testing of the victim. Testing to measure capacity or decisional abilities, an expert may have used instruments such as the Interview for Decisional Abilities (IDA) or Addenbrooke's Cognitive Examinations (ACEs), or, if qualified to do so, may conduct a formal psychiatric evaluation. This type of testing and evaluation, however, may not be available in all communities. In many cases prosecutors rely on the testimony of primary care professionals and APS social workers who may use a general cognitive impairment screening tool such as the Folstein Mini-Mental State Exam (MMSE) [16], the St. Louis University Mental Status (SLUMS) [17] exam or the Montreal Cognitive Assessment (MoCA) [18] to assess a victim along with testimony regarding a victim's cognitive decline from family, friends, acquaintances and family physicians.

In Michael R.'s case, the victim's cognitive decline during the time of the caregiver's employment is a critical issue in determining the scope of the criminal charges. In the early stages of the caregiver's employment, Michael R. gave consent for the caregiver to use one of his debit/credit card accounts to pay for some expenses. None of the spending by the caregiver during this period is criminal since it was prior to Michael R.'s cognitive decline and he gave his knowing consent to the caregiver. During the subsequent years of her employment, however, the caregiver began to spend Michael R.'s assets for her own benefit without his informed consent due to his cognitive decline. It is only this last phase of spending that would be the basis for criminal charges.

While Michael R. did not have a capacity evaluation as part of the case investigation, the trial court allowed other evidence of his cognitive decline to prove the timeline of his impairment. Testimony from Michael R.'s family and associates provided observations regarding his changes in behavior associated with his increasing cognitive issues and his increasing lack of understanding regarding his financial affairs. Michael R.'s son, a physician, testified regarding his cognitive decline. An APS social worker testified that the results of an MMSE screening tool he used to evaluate Michael R. during the period of the exploitation demonstrated cognitive impairment. Michael R.'s long-time primary care physician testified regarding his observations of Michael R.'s cognitive decline over time during office visits and his observations regarding the caregiver's increasing involvement and influence over Michael R.'s decision-making. All this evidence proved essential in establishing the time of the caregiver's criminal financial exploitation of Michael R.

Financial professionals are key witnesses in nearly every elder financial abuse case. A fundamental part of a financial exploitation case is proving the amount of loss and the methods by which the perpetrator took assets belonging to the elder victim. An essential part of that evidence is the complete financial records of the victim and suspect during the relevant time period. Once the records are obtained, they must be entered into software that can produce spreadsheets for analysis. As mentioned earlier in this chapter, most investigators with law enforcement and APS can prepare relatively straightforward financial cases involving limited financial transactions and testify to that work. Law enforcement and APS social workers are not, however, typically trained in organizing large volumes of financial records and analyzing that information to track hundreds of transactions and identify significant changes in the financial positions of the victim and perpetrator over a designated time period. Given the necessity of having such financial information in an understandable format for prosecutors to use in charging decisions and for juries in deciding cases, experts such as forensic accountants or financial analysts are often indispensable and are hired by prosecutors for complex financial cases.

A forensic accountant is typically a licensed certified public accountant, who specializes in financial or accounting fraud investigations. The forensic accountant or financial analyst uses the financial records collected during the investigation to reconstruct past financial events such as a transfer of money to identify whose account the money was transferred from, how it was transferred, and into whose account the money was received. After analyzing the financial records, these financial experts provide expert testimony to the jury to explain the financial transactions at issue and the victim's total loss.

In Michael R.'s case, the prosecutor hired a forensic accountant to assist with the financial aspects of the case because the scope of the records involved multiple years of financial records and multiple financial accounts. The forensic accountant then identified information needed by the prosecutor including the types of transactions the caregiver used to access Michael R.'s assets for her own benefit while he was suffering from cognitive decline and the total amount of loss to Michael R. based on the caregiver's thefts. At trial, the forensic accountant provided critical testimony explaining the hundreds of pages of financial records that had been reviewed and traced each of the transactions so that the jury could understand how the financial records supported the criminal charges filed against the caregiver.

Multi-disciplinary and coordinated responses to elder financial exploitation are central to adequately addressing older victimization. Financial abuse impacts the psychological security of older victims as well as imposing an enormous toll on their economic security. Multi-Disciplinary Teams (MDTs) have been created to provide a coordinated response from professionals to address a victim's needs and security. MDTs include personnel from APS, law enforcement, medical service providers, financial institutions, local aging service agencies and legal and community advocates. The relationships between professionals addressing these difficult cases are strengthened through cooperation and all the members gain a better understanding of the available services that are needed for older adult victims of financial exploitation.

In Michael R.'s case, reports of his abuse were made at a time when there was no MDT in his community. The community, however, received prior federal grant funding for elder abuse training involving prosecutors, law enforcement, and APS that established connections between the professionals and those relationships were instrumental in coordinating the case investigation and in identifying needed services for Michael R. and his family because of the caregiver's abuse.

Key Points

1. Financial exploitation of older adults is devastating to their physical and mental wellbeing. The impact often erodes older adults' self-confidence, decimates their savings, and impairs their ability to live independently.
2. Medical professionals are essential in exposing and acting witnesses in elder financial abuse cases. Because most financial mistreatment cases involve older adults with cognitive impairment, obtaining testimony regarding the cognitive status of a victim is critical in proving whether the suspected financial activity is consensual or if it is criminal.
3. Financial analysts and forensic accountants are essential witnesses in determining the scope of the improper financial transactions that may be criminal and in calculating the financial losses suffered by the older adult.
4. Elder financial mistreatment cases require information from the victim as well as multiple other sources to appropriately address the full impact of the crime—financial, physical, mental—on an older adult.
5. A multidisciplinary perspective—medical, financial, and legal—is needed to uncover areas of financial exploitation that may go undiscovered and thus unresolved. Multi-disciplinary teams (MDTs) are essential in helping to provide and bridge information. Working together, professionals can work quickly to end abuse.

References

1. Lachs M, Han D. Age-associated financial vulnerability: an emerging public health issue. Ann Int Med. 163:877–8.
2. Investor Protection Trust. 2016 website link: https://www.americanbar.org/groups/law_aging/publications/bifocal/vol_38/issue_2_december2015/2016-year-in-review/
3. AARP Bank Safe Initiative: a comprehensive Approach to Better Serving and Protecting Consumers, p. 2 Jan 2016.
4. Elder Abuse.org
5. https://mayoclinic.org
6. Morgan, R Tapp S. Examining financial fraud against older adults. NIJ. March 20, 2024.
7. Wolf RS. Caregiver stress, Alzheimer's disease, and elder abuse. Am J Alzheimers Dis. 1998;13(2):81–3. https://doi.org/10.1177/153331759801300205.
8. Jackson S. All elder abuse perpetrators are not alike: the heterogeneity of elder abuse perpetrators and implications for intervention. Int J Offend Therapy Comp Criminol. 2016;60(3):265–85.
9. Dauenhauer, J., et al. Utilization of a forensic accountant to investigate financial exploitation of older adults. J Adult Prot. 2020;2(3). ISSN 1466–8203.
10. Burnett, J., et al. A collaboration between adult protective services and forensic accounting examiners to investigate complex financial exploitation: formative evaluation findings. J Elder Abuse Negl. 1–18, Published online February 6, 2024. https://doi.org/10.1080/08946566.2024.2315084.
11. Elder Justice Roadmap July 2014.
12. See Stanford Center on Longevity. Framework for a taxonomy of fraud. (12). 2015. https://longevity.stanford.edu/framework-for-a-taxonomy-of-fraud/).
13. https://www.staysafeonline.org/articles/what-is-pig-butchering-and-how-to-spot-the-scam
14. Under the Radar: New York State Elder Abuse Prevalence Study Lifespan of Greater Rochester, p. 50, Weill Cornell Medical (Gunther, AARP. The Thief Who Knows You, Spring 2020).
15. Yaffe MJ, Tazkarii B. Understanding elder abuse in family practice. Can Fam Physician. 2012;58(12):1336–40.
16. Folstein MF, et al. "Mini-mental state": a practice method for grading the cognitive state of patients for the clinician. J Psychiatr Res. 1975;12:189–98.
17. Tariq SH, et al. The Saint Louis University Mental Status (SLUMS) Examination for detecting mild cognitive impairment and dementia is more sensitive than the Mini-M Status Examination (MMSE) a pilot study. Am J Geriatr Psych. 2006;14:900–10.
18. Nasreddine Z, et al. The Montreal Cognitive Assessment MoCA: a brief screening tool for mild cognitive impairment. J Am Geriatr Soc. 2005;53(4):695–9.

Suggested Reading

Mosqueda L, Burnight K, Gironda MW, Moore AA, Robinson J, Olsen B. The Abuse Intervention Model: A Pragmatic Approach to Intervention for Elder Mistreatment. J Am Geriatr Soc. 2016;64(9):1879–83. https://doi.org/10.1111/jgs.14266. Epub 2016 Aug 22. PMID: 27550723; PMCID: PMC5026887.

Chapter 4
Sexual Abuse

Elizabeth M. Bloemen and Sarah Tietz

Introduction

There is substantial evidence that older adults have increasing vulnerability to sexual abuse and assault, particularly if there are risk factors for functional and cognitive impairment such as dementia [1–4]. The majority of older adults who experience sexual violence have cognitive, speech, or functional impairments that limit their ability to report, receive appropriate care, recover from injury, and engage in services. In this population, a specialized approach is critical to minimize the substantial morbidity and mortality that can result from this form of trauma.

Case 1 Presentation

An 84-year-old woman with a past medical history of stroke, hypertension, and seizure disorder presented from her long-term care facility with increased confusion and new bruising. When emergency medical services arrived at the facility she yelled "help me, help me, they hurt me, I went my whole life without this happening." In the emergency department, she was found to have a new ischemic stroke in the left MCA territory and new bruising so the elder abuse team was consulted.

E. M. Bloemen (✉) · S. Tietz
Division of Geriatrics, University of Colorado School of Medicine, Aurora, CO, USA
e-mail: elizabeth.bloemen@cuanschutz.edu

V. LoFaso, L. Rachmuth (eds.), *Elder Abuse and Neglect*,
https://doi.org/10.1007/978-3-031-97784-8_4

On the team's examination her speech was mumbled and tangential and it was difficult to both understand her language. She appeared distressed and continued to express concern about "mean people" and being hurt but wasn't able to give specific details about what occurred. The family reported these as new behaviors and atypical for this patient. The patient's daughter bathed the patient earlier that week and didn't notice any bruising at the time of the bath.

On examination of the skin, circular bruises (~1–3 cm), in linear patterns of 3–4 clustered bruises, in the pattern/size of fingerprints on her bilateral lower extremities in the inner thighs, outer thighs, and inner calves were noted. She had erythema on her right jaw, near her ear. There was also scattered larger bruises seen on her bilateral upper and lower arms, measuring between 5 and 15 cm for each bruise. Smaller bruises were seen on her abdomen and back. An external perineal exam was attempted with family present but terminated early given the victim's significant distress during the exam. During the limited exam, there were no signs of trauma noted to labia minora or majora. Throughout the day, she was willing to participate in routine care, but was very resistant with nursing staff for any perineal care. The team's level of concern was high for sexual abuse but it was not able to be verified given her mental status. STI testing for gonorrhea and chlamydia were able to be obtained through urine sample to avoid the need for vaginal swabs. Evidence collection for semen was unable to be performed. The family declined an exam under anesthesia given low concern for gynecological injury requiring medical intervention.

Case 2 Presentation

An 89 year old male with a history of neurocognitive disorder presents from his long term care facility reporting sexual assault. He is emotionally distressed and reports that someone has hurt him. He is unable to provide details of when, who, or how the assault occurred, but is certain that someone is coming into his room at night to harm him. He reports his concerns are based on the fact that when he wakes in the morning, he will occasionally have a small amount of blood in his undergarments. He reports that this has been going on for years first starting at home, then at his assisted living residence, and now at the skilled nursing facility. On chart review, he has had at least 6 ED visits in the last 2 years with similar reports despite being in different living conditions with different caretakers at each location, and delusional disorder had previously been diagnosed. He reports a history of sexual assault in his teens by a family member. Physical exam is notable for inflammation of the external meatus without any bleeding or excoriations. No rashes or other stigmata of STD's are noted. There was no bruisingor other signs of trauma on exam. The medical provider attempted to reassure him that there weren't signs of sexual assault and that we felt assault was less likely, which resulted in him feeling frustrated, not believed, and like he couldn't trust the medical system.

Sexual Abuse Overview

In older adults with normal cognition, speech, and functional abilities, the assessment and treatment of sexual assault is similar to that for younger victims. However there are some physiologic differences in older adults that should be taken into consideration. For post-menopausal patients, upon examination more lubrication and smaller speculum size should be considered. Other medical conditions may impact mobility and ease of exam (ie chronic pain, arthritis, etc). Co-occurring medical conditions such as atrophic vaginitis or lichen sclerosis can worsen injuries and impair healing. Older adults who are victims of sexual abuse should be tested for STIs, offered treatment and prophylaxis, and provided counseling and resources. Sexual Assault Nurse Examiners and sexual assault advocacy centers are often suitable to address these needs. Advocacy Centers may also assist the victim in reporting the abuse to authorities, depending on the mandatory reporting laws in that state.

Here, we'll discuss some of the more complex scenarios that are seen by specialized hospital based elder abuse teams, discuss our approach of evaluation and management for these patients, and the ethical guidelines for best practices in this complex area of medicine.

Epidemiology and Background

Risk factors for sexual abuse in later life parallel other types of elder abuse including cognitive and functional impairment, dependency on caregivers, social isolation, and prior history of abuse [4].

An important distinction is that the perpetrators of elder sexual violence differ than those of other elder abuse types. Most sexual violence involving family, including "intimate partner violence grown old", is predicated by the need for power and control over the victim. This type of abuse can be more devastating to older victims due to their risk for injury. Older adults may have even more stigma about reporting this type of violence and medical and legal authorities may be less likely to believe victims [1, 5]. Compounding this is a cultural cohort affect as older adults were raised in a period of time when violence within marriage was not necessarily considered illegal or abnormal and therefore may not see sexually violent acts as a form of abuse. There is some literature that sexual violence against older adults may be a form of experimentation or be the result of opportunistic behavior although data supporting this is limited [6, 7]. Because this crime is difficult to identify and prosecute, there are also higher rates and more opportunity for serial perpetration [8].

Reporting in these cases can be exceptionally challenging. Older adults are not generally thought of as sexual beings and this ageist attitude is difficult for most people to grapple with. Medical professionals know many people continue to have consensual sex at all ages.

It is well known that sexual violence is rarely about sexual gratification. The concept of an older adult being sexually assaulted is uncomfortable and disturbing. Due to ageist views and the perception that all older adults have dementia and are unable to report accurately, older victims are often not believed if they report sexual violence [5].

Case 1 Discussion

This patient had cognitive impairment and now has dysarthria and aphasia secondary to her stroke. This patient would ideally see three providers during her care: a forensic or sexual assault nurse examiner, a physician, a geriatrician, and a social worker. Here, we will describe our unique approaches and roles Table 4.1.

Forensic Nurse Approach

Forensic nurse examiners are specially trained and certified to provide care for and collect evidence from victims of violent crimes. A forensic nurse will collect a detailed medical and social history, perform an physical exam, and will collect evidence including clothing, photographs, and swabs of different parts of the body [9, 10]. As in younger patients, older adults who experience sexual assault commonly have no clear injury to the perineum. Absence of visualized injury should not dissuade collection of swabs for evidence.

In post-menopausal women the perineal tissue changes due to the lack of estrogen. The hymen can be particularly sensitive and the tissue is more friable. For this reason we suggest using a pediatric speculum with lubrication for collecting blind

Table 4.1 Recommended Labs and Treatment

Labs:

Sexually transmitted infections:
  Gonorrhea/ chlamydia/trichomonas (consider swabbing any area with a history of penetration including vaginal, rectal, and oropharynx)
  HIV
  Syphilis
Urine toxicology to look for drug facilitated sexual assault

Treatments to consider
Empiric treatment of gonorrhea/ chlamydia Post exposure prophylaxis for HIV HBV vaccination or treatment depending on risk factors of perpetrator and vaccination status of victim Gynecological evaluation if injuries present   Vaginal estrogen may be helpful to help with wound healing if signs of atrophic vaginitis

swabs. While doing the examination the provider should monitor for signs of discomfort and distress. Having a trusted other with the victim can be an option to lend support.

In this case, the practitioners should collect any potential evidence. Appropriate personnel should photograph every bruise and injury. It is essential to document all physical findings, as this information may be pertinent in the future. This patient would not tolerate a speculum exam or blind swabs, so photo documentation and clothing would be the primary sources of evidence collected.

Elder Abuse- Geriatrician Approach

A geriatrician can provide critical, patient-centered care to victims of sexual violence. As this case demonstrates, communicating with patients with cognitive and language impairments is key to understanding what happened and ensuring safety. This patient had a severe stroke, which could be contributing to her emotional lability. She may also have experienced a trauma that could affect her emotional state. Due to common physical changes of aging, it can be challenging to differentiate findings in sexual assault from other medical conditions. In either scenario, this patient is experiencing distress. Responding and validating to what the patient is experiencing is important. In patients with cognitive impairment, psychosis, or other conditions, it can be more distressing if providers try to explain their findings and provide reassurance. Some patients will be unable to process that information. It may make them feel like they aren't believed and their concerns aren't taken seriously [11].

Geriatricians play a crucial role in these cases through trauma-informed capacity assessments. In this case, it was important to assess the victim's ability to consent to the exam and provide evidence to law enforcement. If capacity is in question the patient's Medical Power of attorney should be engaged in decision making [12].

Geriatricians can help interpret injury patterns to better gauge the level of concern for non-accidental trauma. Geriatricians bring expertise in caring for frail older adults with many medical conditions and medications that increase bruising, fractures, and skin breakdown. Ruling out abuse mimics is important and within the purview of a geriatrician. Diseases such as lichen sclerosis, atrophic vaginitis, and cutaneous candidiasis can mimic bruising or injury, and we have seen cases of HSV or zoster that were mistaken as signs of sexual trauma.

The provider is also responsible for ensuring that the appropriate medical care is provided to patients. This includes screening for STIs including gonorrhea, chlamydia, HIV, syphilis, and trichomonas which is routinely considered in younger patients but often overlooked in older adults. If high concern for assault and an unknown perpetrator, post exposure prophylaxis for HIV and empiric treatment for STIs should be considered. It is reasonable to consider vaccination for HBV since many older adults have not previously received vaccination [13].

Social Work Approach

Social workers are a critical component to the response to elder abuse [14]. Social workers provide trauma-informed care to victims and families, support patients in connecting with victim supports and resources, and help with mandatory reporting as well as follow up with police and APS. Reporting for sexual assault cases can require particular sensitivity. Through a psychosocial assessment, a social worker in this case could clarify any points in the history taken by the forensic nurse that may be unclear. If law enforcement is called, it can be helpful to request police officers trained in sexual assault or elder maltreatment, or facilitate an officer of the preferred gender for the patient to improve patient comfort, for example many women will be more comfortable with a woman after a sexual trauma inflicted by a man. Hospital-based social workers can provide victim accompaniment for these interviews, provide emotional support, and help victims be heard. This also presents an opportunity to directly confront ageist assumptions and help victims remain at the center of care and investigations [15].

The social worker can also provide brief therapy and connection to resources in the community. Community resources can be somewhat challenging to find for older victims, but sexual assault advocacy centers can be a good place to start. In most cases, adult protective services will also be engaged and can providing ongoing care and support in the community.

Case 2 Discussion

Delusions are a common symptom of neurocognitive disorders and can be a primary presenting symptom of dementia. Delusions in older adults should be treated similarly to younger adults, by excluding all other etiologies and providing empathetic care that does not directly challenge the delusion. It is important to not assume that reports of sexual assault in older adults with dementia are delusions, reports should be made, and the proper investigative agencies should be involved. Those with a history of trauma and a history of neurocognitive disorders are more likely to experience sexual abuse in later age. However, we have seen a number of cases where patients have delusions of sexual assault which was confirmed after reports were made and police were able to investigate video footage to confirm no one entered that person's room during the evening of the report. Often these patients will have repeated presentations after thorough investigation by APS and law enforcement without findings of abuse occurring. These repeated reports and presentations are often distressing and frustrating to patients who feel dismissed and not believed.

The patients that we most commonly see with this type of delusion often experienced sexual trauma earlier in life. And that person often was not believed or supported when they reported their prior abuse in earlier life, compounding the challenge of supporting these patients when we are uncertain that abuse has occurred recently. These are often very distressing to patients and supportive care is very important. Providers should communicate level of concern to investigators but provide support to the patient and not counter their delusion. The experience of the delusion is as distressing to each person as a validated sexual assault and support should be provided with a similar rigor. These patients are also ideal victims and can be targets for violence, so future reports should always be taken seriously and attended to regardless of the history of delusions. We recommend offering sample collection, and repeating STI testing as it is a low risk intervention and the risk of missing an infection can cause harm to a patient.

This case also highlights that medical conditions can often mimic findings we see in sexual abuse. Atrophic vaginitis caused perineal discomfort and perineal bleeding which can often be confused for signs of assault by both patients and medical providers alike. We recommended treatment with a vaginal estrogen ring that could be replaced every 3 months to help prevent bleeding and discomfort. The ring (versus estrogen cream) also allowed application every 3 months instead of multiple times weekly to help decrease distress for this patient.

Key Points

1. Believe victims: Sexual assault in later life happens. Victims are often not believed due to ageism and a belief that older adults are not sexual beings. Additionally, most providers are distressed at the thought that an older adult may have been sexually assaulted and this distress can lead providers to search for other possible reasons for a presentation. While alternative etiologies for an exam finding are always important to consider, believing victims and considering sexual assault as an etiology is important.
2. Make sure older adults get the appropriate treatment: STI testing and treatment, special consideration for increased risk of HBV given vaccine history and HIV given fragility of perineal tissues. When in doubt treat empirically!
3. Trauma informed examination in the setting of cognitive impairment is very important and should be based on the experience of the patient, not necessarily substantiated abuse.
4. Capacity evaluation around reporting, consenting to exam, consenting vs assenting to sexual activity needs to be undertaken and if a patient lacks capacity and appropriate decision maker should be engaged in care.
5. Mimics of sexual abuse can include lichen, zoster, atrophic vaginitis, candidiasis, medical devices (foley, rectal tube, etc), and other infections and should be thoroughly considered and treated.

6. Geriatricians can often play a key role by educating adult protective services and law enforcement officers about cognitive deficits and providing patient support during interview
7. Unfortunately, many victims experience sexual assault earlier in life and this can manifest in the course of their neurocognitive disorder. Delusions related to sexual assault should remain a diagnosis of exclusion and support should be provided to patients.
8. Caring for victims of sexual assault across the lifecourse can be distressing to providers, and this distress can be amplified when older adults are involved. This distress combined with entrenched ageism can cause providers to want to find any other reason for a patient's presentation other than an assault, but unfortunately sexual assault in later life does happen. Providing support to both patients and those involved in their care is important to ensure that everyone can live free from abuse.

References

1. Nobels A, Keygnaert I, Robert E, et al. 'Breaking the silence': sexual victimisation in an old age psychiatry patient population in Flanders. Int J Geriatr Psychiatry. 2021;36(10):1550–8.
2. Smith D, Cunningham N, Willoughby M, et al. The epidemiology of sexual assault of older female nursing home residents, in Victoria Australia, between 2000 and 2015. Leg Med (Tokyo, Japan). 2019;36:89–95.
3. Lee JA, Majeed-Ariss R, Pedersen A, Yusuf F, White C. Sexually assaulted older women attending a U.K. sexual assault referral centre for a forensic medical examination. J Forensic Leg Med. 2019;68:101859.
4. Cannell MB, Manini T, Spence-Almaguer E, Maldonado-Molina M, Andresen EM. U.S. population estimates and correlates of sexual abuse of community-dwelling older adults. J Elder Abuse Negl. 2014;26(4):398–413.
5. Band-Winterstein T, Goldblatt H, Lev S. Breaking the taboo: sexual assault in late life as a multifaceted phenomenon-toward an integrative theoretical framework. Trauma Violence Abuse. 2021;22(1):112–24.
6. Georgoulis H, Beauregard E, Chopin J. A criminological perspective on the sexual victimization of older adults. Curr Psychiatry Rep. 2024;26(3):53–9.
7. Chopin J, Beauregard E. Sexual abuse of elderly victims investigated by the police: from motives to crime characteristics. J Interpers Violence. 2021;36(13–14):6722–44.
8. Speck PM, Hartig MT, Likes W, et al. Case series of sexual assault in older persons. Clin Geriatr Med. 2014;30(4):779–806.
9. Burgess AW, Hanrahan NP, Baker T. Forensic markers in elder female sexual abuse cases. Clin Geriatr Med. 2005;21(2):399–412.
10. Hargot LA. The sexual assault examination. Can Fam Physician. 1985;31:775–80.
11. Bloemen EM, Tietz S, Lindberg DM, Hayes J, Lum H, Gottesman E, Elman A, Sullivan M, Pino C, McAuley J, Shaw A, Hancock D, Chang E-S, Yasui R, LoFaso VM, Stern ME, Rosen T. Elder abuse geriatrics: describing an important new medical specialist. J Elder Abuse Negl. 2024;36(4):367–83.
12. Bloemen EM, Gottesman E, Furfari K, et al. Examining ethical issues that arise in providing ED/hospital care for patients experiencing elder mistreatment and approaches to address them. J Elder Abuse Negl. 2024;36(4):395–412.

13. Workowski KA, Bachmann LH, Chan PA, et al. Sexually transmitted infections treatment guidelines, 2021. MMWR Recomm Rep. 2021;70(4):1–187.
14. Elman A, Cox S, Gottesman E, et al. The critical role of the specialized social worker as part of ED/hospital-based elder mistreatment response teams. J Elder Abuse Negl. 2024;36(4):1–11.
15. Goldblatt H, Band-Winterstein T, Lev S, Harel D. "Who would sexually assault an 80-year-old woman?": Barriers to exploring and exposing sexual assault against women in late life. J Interpers Violence. 2022;37(5–6):2751–75.

Chapter 5
Emotional Abuse

Dina Patel and Elaine Suben

Introduction

Emotional abuse is a highly prevalent form of elder abuse resulting in significant pain and suffering for the victim. Characterized by threats, humiliation, intimidation and isolation, this form of abuse can lead to long-lasting adverse psychological and physical sequelae. Emotional abuse is often perpetrated by individuals close to the victim, most commonly spouses or adult children and can leave the victim feeling powerless and depressed. It is important that health care and other service providers consider this form of abuse whenever an older adult presents with an unexplained change in their physical or emotional status.

Case Presentation

DR is a 72-year-old Latin American, cis gendered female, married, religious catholic, domiciled. She has not worked for many decades and is financially dependent on her husband of 50 years. She is Medicaid eligible. Her family resides in the Bronx in New York City. Until recently, her granddaughter lived with them, and was very involved in her care. Due to a debilitating diagnosis of rheumatoid arthritis DR was reliant on her granddaughter for some ADL's (bathing, transferring) and some

D. Patel (✉)
Gramercy Psychiatry and Weill Cornell Medicine, New York, NY, USA
e-mail: dap9153@med.cornell.edu

E. Suben
The Center on Aging, NY Presbyterian Hospital, New York, NY, USA

V. LoFaso, L. Rachmuth (eds.), *Elder Abuse and Neglect*,
https://doi.org/10.1007/978-3-031-97784-8_5

IADL's (cooking and medication management). After her granddaughter left, she had to again rely on her husband to carry out these tasks.

In a recent appointment to her primary care physician, she was noted to be more disheveled, avoiding eye contact and appearing sad. Her primary care physician asked about her wellbeing, and she burst into tears. However, when asked to discuss what was happening, she was unable to articulate her feelings. The PCP referred her to a clinical social worker who is part of the interdisciplinary collaborative care team for counseling. Patient was then referred to a psychiatrist for further evaluation.

On evaluation with the psychiatrist, she admitted to feeling lonely since her granddaughter moved out. Her granddaughter was not only a great help physically but also a companion. Her adult children are unfortunately in other states and unable to assist. She notes that since her granddaughter moved out, she has not been able to care for herself as well. When asked about support from her husband, she appears withdrawn, becomes quieter, and states "I don't know". After some discussion, she discloses that her husband has been increasingly aggressive, threatening to withhold her meals if she doesn't "shut up", at times withholding her pain medication as punishment if he feels she is asking for too much assistance. She further reveals he had been hurting her both emotionally and physically since they were married, however more recently emotional abuse was dominant.

She would cope in the past by going to her church and being around other family members. Whenever she would leave the house, he would always ask her where she was going and often accuse her of seeing other men, calling her names, swearing at her, saying no one wants to talk to someone stupid like her. It was often worse when he would be drinking. Although he would be this way with her behind closed doors, when others were around he would be able to switch to a charming man. She did not see the point of telling anyone the truth, and felt that if she did, people may not believe her or may justify that this is normal. When asking more about how this could be perceived as normal, she revealed that she had also grown up witnessing her parents fight both physically and emotionally for many years. She felt guilt and shame even talking about all this now. She laments no longer being physically healthy enough to go out of the house on her own and misses church and friends.

More recently with worsening rheumatoid arthritis and her granddaughter moving out, she has become more isolated, and more often alone with her husband without reprieve. Her husband does not allow non-family members in the house, so she has not been able to get an aide for assistance despite qualifying. And since her granddaughter moved out, she must rely on him for all assistance. She has difficulty with ADL's, including walking without assistance, reaching for high objects, showering, and more. Recently she has given up on some of these things in lieu of angering her husband if she asked for help.

She also notes recurrence of symptoms she had in her childhood - nightmares, panic attacks, avoidance, hypervigilance. These symptoms of PTSD have been increasing since her granddaughter left and she experiences additional symptoms of low mood, fear, and at times hopelessness. She always believed her symptoms were "nerves" and that there wasn't much to do about it. She was raised to also keep personal problems to herself. She recognizes in the session that she needs help now but has no idea how to access it.

Emotional Abuse Overview

Psychological abuse has several risk factors, including prior depression, anxiety, cognitive impairment, loneliness, dependent personality, and functional dependency [8, 9]. Psychological distress is also a risk factor manifesting even more in individuals with lower socioeconomic status [9].

Common stress reactions can include: rage, fear, nightmares, tearfulness, night terrors, depression, sadness; physical reactions: numbness, fatigue, physical pain, rapid heart rate and breathing, tight muscles, sleep problems; thinking reactions (paranoia and dissociation) and behavioral reactions (irritability, withdrawal, reactivity, violence) [10, 11]. Stress can negatively impact cognition, memory, and aging, and repeated trauma can have compounding effects on an individuals functional ability [11]. Verbal abuse (name calling, yelling, demeaning and threatening) is another method the alleged perpetrator uses to chisel away at the victim's self-esteem, leaving them in a vulnerable and hostile situation. It is imperative to consider these risk factors in everyday evaluation of older adults as there is a unique opportunity for clinicians to intervene with education before mistreatment occurs.

After emotional abuse occurs there are inevitably psychological consequences. Most notably the victim is at risk for new onset or recurrence of depression, anxiety, and PTSD [12–14]. Other responses are fear, guilt, shame, learned helplessness, and withdrawal. As one can imagine, the psychological impact will in turn affect physical health as evidenced by-decreased adherence to medication and nutrition as victims become overwhelmed. Although emotional abuse may be less obvious as physical abuse, it can be just as detrimental.

Case Discussion

Several risk factors for emotional abuse are highlighted in DR's case: (1) intimate partner violence, including physical and emotional/verbal abuse throughout the course of their 50 year relationship (2) chronic debilitating medical conditions including rheumatoid arthritis (3) diagnosis of PTSD, depression and anxiety (4) lack of social support systems, low income/socioeconomic status, social isolation (5) "toxic stress"- ongoing and relentless body responses to intense stressors (6) prolonged activation of her stress response systems in the absence of a protective relationship (7) cognitive impairment and (8) dependent personality [15].

She meets criteria for PTSD, and given her tearful presentation on examination with evidence of low mood, she would warrant further evaluation to assess for

Major Depressive Disorder and suicidality. Of note, a study of depressed elder abuse victims found PTSD to be in more than half of the sample, with higher reported rates in those that experienced emotional mistreatment versus physical mistreatment [16]. These individuals with PTSD also had a higher rate of suicidal ideation. Intervention with a brief therapy called PROTECT resulted in reductions in symptoms. PROTECT, which stands for Providing Options to Elderly Clients Together, involved therapists going to a clients home and providing practical and evidence based mental health interventions. This study clearly demonstrates the importance of not only assessing for PTSD in older adults who experienced elder abuse, but also ruling out or treating suicidal ideation, given its high prevalence in this population.

Additionally, DR's expression of fear should prompt a complete evaluation for symptoms of anxiety. She uses the word "normal" to describe her symptoms, so careful education on symptoms related to anxiety, depression and PTSD may help her regain agency. Learned helplessness is common in this population and may prevent individuals from seeking assistance. It is beneficial to normalize that guilt, shame, and withdrawal are common reactions to the stressful experiences.

Human beings thrive on social connection within a framework of social systems of support. When one is deprived of interactions within one's community, serious psychological damage can occur. Trust is broken and a sense of safety and security is violated in the wake of emotional abuse. Stressors experienced in the present can trigger associations or traumatic memories of the past. By socially isolating DR, her husband exerts his power and control. "Lack of social connection is as dangerous as smoking 15 cigarettes a day." [17] As DR becomes more socially isolated she experiences a constant state of hypervigilance that may result in social withdrawal for self-protection and difficulty forming positive relationships [18, 19]. This hypervigilance can affect cognition and perception as the brain is on high alert [19].

DR's granddaughter had to disengage from the daily care of her grandmother due to her own health problems. DR's care is now in the hands of her husband, thereby increasing her dependence on him, and further deepening the emotional wounds already inflicted on her throughout their relationship. DR reports she is experiencing frequent nightmares resulting in poor quality of sleep and an increase in anxiety. In addition, the victim's physical health is declining resulting in loss of independence, mobility, and self-determination.

The case of DR sheds light on the intricacies of a case of psychological abuse in elder mistreatment. Viewing the case from a biopsychosocial perspective gives insight into the multiple facets of emotional abuse. The theories of domestic abuse (intimate partner violence), intergenerational transmission of violence, and abuse across the lifespan can help one conceptualize what DR is experiencing.

One theory of domestic abuse is *the power and control theory*, which posits that there is an imbalance of power where one partner dominates the other most commonly the male dominating the female. Due to traditional gender roles, the power dynamic is such that women are blamed for the abuse and often in turn blame themselves. In this theory the man uses coercive tactics to maintain this control, including physical and verbal abuse. We can see in this case, her husband maintains power through his aggression, withholding medication, and his threats [3, 4].

Intergenerational transmission of violence, a part of social learning theory, can explain why DR felt some of what she experienced was “normal”. In this theory, children who witness violence in their childhood learn that violence is a way to interact and then imitate this action. As they grow up, they may continue to use violence in their relationship or view this as part of acceptable behavior. In this case it may be that DR’s husband had experienced this in his childhood in addition to DR experiencing this within her family [5].

Another consideration is that domestic abuse in younger years continues into adulthood. Domestic violence is cyclical, often repeating throughout the lifetime, which is known as abuse across the lifespan. As mentioned by DR, her husband was abusive early in their marriage, both emotionally and physically. Although it seems that the physical abuse lessened, the emotional abuse accelerated [6].

Finally, the alleged abuser may also have his/her own risk factors to consider, such as mental health conditions, substance use, and type of upbringing [7]. Risk factors for becoming a perpetrator include mental illness, substance abuse, caregiver stress, previous history of family violence, and financial dependence on older adults.

Careful history taking, observation of mood and engagement, and understanding risk factors of an older adult can uncover elder abuse. Survivors of elder abuse can benefit from “short term planning, long term counseling, and ongoing supportive services” which helps increase self-esteem and coping mechanisms [2].

DR is receiving ongoing psychiatric support via weekly psychotherapy sessions and monthly medication management for depressive symptoms. Her PCP referred her for a biopsychosocial assessment by a social worker to obtain additional support within the framework of trauma informed care.

The initial meeting would ideally take place in a private office setting to facilitate calm and a sense of safety and well-being. It may begin with an introduction to relaxation and breathing techniques to activate the parasympathetic nervous system to produce the “rest and digest” response and reduce hyperarousal [20]. Social workers are trained to ‘meet the client where she is’, to promote the client’s agency and self-determination, and to assess DR’s readiness to disclose her story, accepting help is essential. Utilizing a strengths-based approach, we can identify what is working for DR and how she can build from there to increase confidence and move toward her goals. With this approach there is less pathologizing of her experience and more emphasis on positive steps towards healing and wellness [21].

The initial encounter should allow for choice, collaboration, trustworthiness, and empowerment, and provide a safe, welcoming, and supportive space [22]. Meet the victim where she is and ask permission to inquire about sensitive issues. The interview should proceed slowly and with caution so as not to re-traumatize. The interviewer should offer breaks from intense discussions and provide support and empathic listening. A skilled clinician will be mindful of DR’s cues and normalize her feelings. Screening for trauma and providing psychoeducation about emotional abuse can promote agency in seeking treatment options. Connecting DR to appropriate resources (from organizations/providers with trauma informed practices) and developing a treatment plan collaboratively with DR incorporating what matters most to her and will increase engagement and adherence to a plan. Both parties (patient and clinician) recognize that establishing rapport and a therapeutic alliance takes time and consistency; set expectations (frequency and method of communication with clinician) and establish and maintain "healthy boundaries". Healthy boundaries include appropriateness of clinician's self-disclosure, awareness of body language, and adequate spatial distancing while in session, and adherence to schedules (start and stop appts on time) [23]. Boundaries provide a framework to ensure the protection of the victim and avoidance of burnout and secondary traumatization of the clinician [23]. Finally, reinforce DR's strengths by reviewing her progress and the steps she has taken to obtain support using affirmative and empowering language.

Approach the individual with sensitivity and be sure to understand the victim's feelings regarding both the perpetraor and abuse [2]. This is accomplished via engagement, rapport and trust building, and normalization and validation of her experience and feelings. Psycho-education about elder abuse and mistreatment is equally as important as safety planning. Safety planning is a personalized plan done in advance to improve safety while experiencing, planning to leave, or after leaving, an abusive situation as it may be hard to think clearly when in crisis [21].

In addressing the needs of a mistreated older adult it is prudent to use trauma informed care. The skilled clinician recognizes the impact of traumatic experiences on the victim's current functioning and makes every effort to listen, support and reflect back with gentle responses and interventions that are sensitively timed to alleviate fear and distrust [24]. On a broader systems level, it behooves institutions, facilities and clinics that serve older adults who may have experienced trauma to integrate environments that are welcoming and inclusive, and provide their healthcare professionals with policies that promote work-life balance and physical and emotional well- being.

While our focus is predominantly on DR, assessing the abuser's willingness to change is also crucial. Try connecting the perpetrator to mandated or voluntary group or individual psychotherapy, counseling, rehabilitation, or anger management services, such as batterer intervention programs. It is important to know that victims "often come forward for the sake of the abuser", creating an opportunity for intervention [2]. Additionally, referral to caregiver resources, for example caregiver support groups and respite care, can be helpful in cases with where overwhelming caregiving needs may be contributing to the abuse.

Role of Psychiatry and Social Work

A biopsychosocial evaluation is often used in these cases. Addressing biological, psychological, and social components is key to understanding and unraveling the complexity of what is seen in elder abuse cases. This evaluation includes presenting and personal history, medical, mental health and substance use history, as well as family history, employment, and education.

Start by meeting the victim where she is; build rapport, trust and therapeutic alliance. What is the timeline of events that are relevant? Be sure to identify severity and frequency of symptoms and triggers of symptoms as well as assess strengths and motivation for treatment. Outline the current challenges that the patient is facing – for example, what brings her to seek treatment at this point in time as versus a year ago, have they taken steps to address the abuse, are there safety concerns?

Clarify the personal history, in particular place of birth, immigration status, composition of family of origin (parents and siblings) and extended family, sexual orientation and gender identity, social supports (including primary supports), educational background, cultural influences, spiritual and religious affiliations, interests and hobbies. Describe work history, career and educational goals/experiences; was the victim financially independent in the past; if so how has that changed? Are there family of origin dynamics to be considered that may provide context; has the victim witnessed or been exposed to violence as a younger person; are there genetic or environmental factors that may contribute to vulnerability of the victim? This information is key in understanding who the person is and ultimately allowing the clinician to best gear treatment for the individual.

Assess for the patient's risk level by understanding prior psychiatric treatment, including hospitalizations, suicide attempts, prior or current psychotherapy. It is helpful to know the dates and location, course of treatment, length of stay of any prior inpatient admissions. Inquire about family history of medical, mental health or substance abuse disorders. How might this influence their current state from a biological, psychological or social standpoint? What is the victim's current relationship to substances (alcohol, illicit drugs, tobacco)? Has the victim struggled with addiction in the past and if so how long was she in recovery?

After a complete assessment, psychiatry would then formulate a treatment plan and provide ongoing supportive counseling and medication management as indicated. Collaboration with social work for support and accessing resources would be an important additional component of care.

Given the complex nature of elder abuse and the multidimensional needs and problems of victims, the use of a multidisciplinary team (MDT) approach is the recommended gold standard for interventions. As Blowers et al. state: "detecting and preventing elder mistreatment requires the involvement of professionals and community partners from many disciplines. It is a community problem, a legal issue, a social concern, and a medical matter." [25, 26].

Advocates and counselors of victims of domestic violence, as well as legal and medical professionals, need to assess their client's emotional state to prevent further traumatization. Efforts to empower the individual to make her own decisions should be the priority. Allowing a woman to choose promotes the healing process and restores power and control. Mills argues that each case is individual and that no one formula for intervention is right for all victims. She advocates that professionals working with domestic violence victims obtain specialized training so that they can recognize the impact of trauma on their clients and themselves [27].

Role of Medical Provider

A primary care physician would do a careful review of the victim's overall health including chronic medical conditions and access to healthcare services. Understanding that elder abuse victims often fail to attend routine medical screenings and preventative measures, the physician would inquire about health maintenance lapses (such as vaccines and cancer screening) and educate the patient about the importance of regular health visits. Making scheduled visits with her PCP at regular interval would allow for assessment of physical or mental decline, and for interventions should they be necessary. Understanding the role of chronic stress on health outcomes and educating the patient about strategies to reduce stress would be a major focus. Along with psychiatry, addressing mental health concerns would also be crucial. Encouraging exercise, good nutrition, and social connection, as well as letting the patient know you are available for check-ins, can strengthen the doctor-patient alliance.

Barriers to Care

It is important to consider what health disparities and/or barriers DR may have faced as a female Latina living and working in the US. Elder abuse affects Latin Americans disproportionally, and they report experiencing discrimination in healthcare more frequently than white individuals. Being born in the United States or holding a college degree does not appear to protect them from such treatment [28]. Additionally, DR had lost her main social support. Individuals and groups who are socially isolated may be more vulnerable to unjust and prejudicial treatment [17]

Race is an example of social determinants of health (SDOH), a major contributor to barriers to care. SDOH is defined as the "conditions that exist in the environments where people are born, live, learn, work, play, worship, and age that affect a wide range of health, functioning, and quality of life outcomes and risks" [Social Determinants of Health and Older Adults. Social Determinants of health and older adults. (2025, March 17). https://odphp.health.gov/our-work/national-health-initiatives/healthy-aging/social-determinants-health-and-older-adults]. Examples of SDOHs are safe housing, racism, discrimination and violence, education, job opportunities, and access to nutritious food [29]. As clinicians we can use strategies to combat this.

Providers should enter the relationship with curiosity and eagerness to learn about a client's culture: customs, traditions, holiday celebrations, cuisine and music. One can ask about language preference for communication and if she prefers a translator to be present. Also be sure to explore one's own explicit and implicit biases [30]. In providing care for patients of minority populations, maintain an awareness of racial, ethnic and cultural differences. Keep in mind how power dynamics within a clinician/patient relationship impact the victim's experience and sense of agency and self-determination. As of 2021, the American Psychological Association (APA) reported that approximately 80.85% of the psychology workforce in the United

States was made up of white professionals [31]. There is a scarcity of mental health clinicians of color which deter BIPOC individuals from seeking services, as they may not identify with or see a likeness of themselves in the provider.

Being mindful of these hurdles can help clinicians break through the barriers. For example, social work can employ this concept in assessing DR's access and connection to services such as healthcare, legal, social service resources, elder abuse mistreatment and prevention programs, older adult socialization programs, and case management. Make every effort to stand up against social injustice to eliminate healthcare disparities and promote access to support and services. Advocacy is key.

Gender

In relation to their male counterparts, women are more likely to be vulnerable due to economic and social factors [32]. As such, they may need to stay with their male partners despite safety concerns. This vulnerability is intensified by chronic medical conditions, inequality, mental health concerns, and aging. Women of color are disproportionately affected by emotional elder abuse, as healthcare disparities impact connecting to services [33].

Ageism

Society's ageist views assign more power to younger individuals and views older individuals as inferior. Older adults can be less valued, often seen as contributing less, when in fact they are able to contribute in both tangible and intangible ways. For example, it is not unusual for older adults to continue working, volunteering, mentoring, and learning. However, ageism relies on the stereotype that older adults are unable to do things, are weak, and are reliant. Family of origin and culture does contribute, as individualistic societies value older adults less than community-based cultures. Even at a young age, one formulates the concept of aging based on what is reflected by their family, society, and community. Licensed professionals including doctors, lawyers, and social workers, are in the position to advocate for the needs of older adults to ensure that they are not mistreated or abused. Utilizing a team approach we can speak up for vulnerable older adults and work towards changing ageist and discriminatory policies or systems that perpetuate oppression and silence their voices [34].

Ethical Dilemmas

Many professions are governed by a code of ethics, which includes a set of practice guidelines and moral principles. These are designed to ensure that those we serve are treated equitably and fairly, and that those in power do not misuse their authority to jeopardize the health and well-being of individuals in their care. The core values of the social work practice are "service, social justice, dignity and worth of a person, importance of human relationships, integrity and competence" [35].

Differences in decision-making and core values may exist across professionals involved in an elder abuse case. These professionals vary in approach and services. For example, DR may disclose facts about the abuse to her internist who then may not have had the time and resources to pass this information to a psychiatrist, which then could undermine the care plan. Her psychiatrist may uncover patterns of emotional abuse inflicted on DR by the perpetrator but due to doctor-patient confidentiality and the victim's right to self-determination, that abuse may go unreported to legal counsel or law enforcement. Preserving the dignity and worth of a victim of elder emotional abuse by exploring the advantages and risks of disclosing the abuse, as opposed to mandating the disclosure, may empower DR to make decisions that promote her safety and resilience. Unlike laws that are enforceable and concrete, ethical issues are not legally enforceable and can be abstract or unwritten.

Respect for confidentiality and trust is integral in cases where serious harm is caused however, the professional may disclose information without obtaining consent. For example, the clinician may experience a dilemma between reporting to APS versus protecting DR's privacy. Another conflict could be encouraging DR to leave and go somewhere safe versus respecting her autonomy. Social workers face a decision-making challenge: to refrain from intervention or try to prevent harm - beneficence vs nonmaleficence [36].

Treatment Plan

A treatment plan is the framework for goals and objectives for the victim. The victim is an active participant in creating a treatment plan with the provider. The treatment plan states the presenting problems. For example: DR is a victim of emotional elder abuse and suffers symptoms of PTSD, depression and anxiety.

A. Treatment Goals

   1. Reduce severity and frequency of symptoms
   2. Develop coping strategies to reduce impact of symptoms on current functioning

B. Treatment objectives

   1. DR to attend monthly medication management appointments with psychiatrist
   2. DR to access social work services to increase support
   3. DR to engage in weekly psychotherapy sessions to explore ways to improve self-esteem and promote wellbeing
   4. Assist DR to formulate a Safety Plan (strategies for where to go and what to do if crisis occurs)

C. Recommendations

DR has several strengths, as she is intelligent and motivated for treatment. She will benefit from ongoing mental health treatment and social services support to reduce the impact of stressors and increase coping mechanisms.

She also would benefit from Adult Protective Services, or APS. APS is part of the social work team. They provide state-mandated services for individuals 18 years of age and older. To qualify for APS services the individual must be mentally or physically impaired and unable to carry out ADLs or protect themselves from abuse and have no one available who is willing and able to assist. Services include referrals for psychiatric and medical examinations and ongoing care, access to government benefits/entitlements, guardianship proceedings, home health care, eviction prevention, and heavy duty cleaning.

Key Points

1. Emotional abuse often coexists with other types of abuse (ex: physical, financial etc)
2. Abuse across the lifespan occurs, and repeated trauma can result in iPTSD, depression and anxiety as well as other negative physical health effects
3. Respecting the victims' right to self-determination should be a guiding principle
4. Social determinants of health and intersectionality (gender, socioeconomic status, race, ethnicity, age) are important considerations in elder abuse
5. Ageism is a significant driver of elder abuse and providers should be aware of ageist attitudes in themselves and society at large
6. Trauma informed care can be helpful in building a therapeutic alliance
7. A multidisciplinary approach is required to address complex issues
8. Despite caregiving stress, the majority of caregivers experiencing stress do not perpetrate abuse
9. Respite care for the caregiver when appropriate can diffuse stressful and potentially harmful family dynamics

References

1. https://dictionary.apa.org/emotional-abuse
2. Breckman RS, Adelman RD, University of Michigan School of Social Work. Strategies for helping victims of elder mistreatment. Newbury Park: Sage Publications; 1988.
3. Walsh CA, Ploeg J, Lohfeld L, Horne J, MacMillan H, Lai D. Violence across the lifespan: interconnections among forms of abuse as described by marginalized Canadian elders and their care-givers. Br J Soc Work. 2007;37(3):491–514. https://doi.org/10.1093/bjsw/bcm022.
4. Brandl B. Power and control: understanding domestic abuse in later life. Generations. 2000;24(2):39–45. JSTOR, http://www.jstor.org/stable/44878440. Accessed 10 May 2024.
5. Hyde-Nolan ME, Juliao T. Theoretical basis for family violence. In: Fife RS, Scharger S, editors. Family violence: what health care providers need to know. Ontario: Jones & Bartlett Learning; 2012. p. 5–16.

6. Symes L. Abuse across the lifespan: prevalence, risk, and protective factors. Nurs Clin North Am. 2011;46(4):391–411. https://doi.org/10.1016/j.cnur.2011.08.008. Epub 2011 Oct 6. PMID: 22055897.
7. Rosen T, Stern ME, Elman A, Mulcare MR. Identifying and initiating intervention for elder abuse and neglect in the emergency department. Clin Geriatr Med. 2018;34(3):435–51. https://doi.org/10.1016/j.cger.2018.04.007.
8. Acierno R, Hernandez-Tejada MA, Anetzberger GJ, Loew D, Muzzy W. The National Elder Mistreatment Study: An 8-year longitudinal study of outcomes. J Elder Abuse Negl. 2017;29(4):254–69.
9. Dong X, Simon MA, Gorbien M, Percak J, Golden R. Loneliness in older Chinese adults: a risk factor for elder mistreatment. J Am Geriatr Soc. 2007;55:1831–5.
10. Bucci M, Marques SS, Oh D, Harris NB. Toxic stress in children and adolescents. Adv Pediatr Infect Dis. 2016;63(1):403–28. https://doi.org/10.1016/j.yapd.2016.04.002. PMID: 27426909.
11. Lupien SJ, McEwen BS, Gunnar MR, Heim C. Effects of stress throughout the lifespan on the brain, behaviour and cognition. Nat Rev Neurosci. 2009;10(6):434–45. https://doi.org/10.1038/nrn2639. Epub 2009 Apr 29. PMID: 19401723.
12. Fisher BS, Regan SL. The extent and frequency of abuse in the lives of older women and their relationship with health outcomes. Gerontologist. 2006;46(2):200–9. https://doi.org/10.1093/geront/46.2.200. PMID: 16581884.
13. Comijs HC, Penninx BW, Knipscheer KP, van Tilburg W. Psychological distress in victims of elder mistreatment: the effects of social support and coping. J Gerontol B Psychol Sci Soc Sci. 1999;54(4):P240–5. https://doi.org/10.1093/geronb/54b.4.p240. PMID: 12382593.
14. Dong XQ, Chen RJ, Chang E-S, Simon M. Elder abuse and psychological well-being: a systematic review and implications for research and policy - a mini review. Gerontology. 2013;59(2):132–42. https://doi.org/10.1159/000341652.
15. Shonkoff JP, Thomas Boyce W, McEwen BS. Neuroscience, molecular biology, and the childhood roots of health disparities: building a new framework for health promotion and disease prevention. JAMA. 2009;301(21):2252–9. Web.
16. Sirey J, Scher C, Solomonov N. PTSD among elder abuse victims with depressed mood. Innov Aging. 2018;2(suppl_1):989. https://doi.org/10.1093/geroni/igy031.3657.
17. Office of the Surgeon General (OSG). Our epidemic of loneliness and isolation: The U.S. Surgeon General's Advisory on the Healing Effects of Social Connection and Community [Internet]. Washington (DC): US Department of Health and Human Services; 2023.
18. Lieberz J, Shamay-Tsoory SG, Saporta N, Esser T, Kuskova E, Stoffel-Wagner B, Hurlemann R, Scheele D. Loneliness and the social brain: how perceived social isolation impairs human interactions. Adv Sci. 2021;8:2102076. https://doi.org/10.1002/advs.202102076.
19. Cacioppo S, Capitanio JP, Cacioppo JT. Toward a neurology of loneliness. Psychol Bull. 2014;140(6):1464–504. https://doi.org/10.1037/a0037618. Epub 2014 Sep 15. PMID: 25222636; PMCID: PMC5130107.
20. LeBouef T, Yaker Z, Whited L. Physiology, autonomic nervous system. [Updated 2023 May 1]. In: StatPearls [Internet]. Treasure Island (FL): StatPearls Publishing; 2024 Jan-. Available from: https://www.ncbi.nlm.nih.gov/books/NBK538516/
21. Sabri B, Tharmarajah S, Njie-Carr VPS, Messing JT, Loerzel E, Arscott J, Campbell JC. Safety planning with marginalized survivors of intimate partner violence: challenges of conducting safety planning intervention research with marginalized women. Trauma Violence Abuse. 2022;23(5):1728–51. https://doi.org/10.1177/15248380211013136. Epub 2021 May 6. PMID: 33955283; PMCID: PMC8571112.
22. Harris M, Fallot RD, editors. Using trauma theory to design service systems. New directions for mental health services. San Francisco: Jossey-Bass; 2001.
23. Editor to help citation: https://www.therapistaid.com/therapy-worksheet/boundaries-psychoeducation-printout

24. Menschner C, Maul A, Center for Health Care Strategies, Inc, Robert Wood Johnson Foundation. Key ingredients for successful trauma-informed care implementation. Trenton/Princeton: Center for Health Care Strategies, Inc./Robert Wood Johnson Foundation; 2016.
25. Blowers A, Davis B, Shenk D, Kalaw KJ, Smith M, Jackson K. A multidisciplinary approach to detecting and responding to elder mistreatment: creating a University-community partnership. Am J Crim Justice. 2012;37:276–90. https://doi.org/10.1007/s12103-012-9156-4.
26. Van Royen K, Van Royen P, De Donder L, Gobbens RJ. Elder abuse assessment tools and interventions for use in the home environment: a scoping review. Clin Interv Aging. 2020;15:1793–807. https://doi.org/10.2147/CIA.S261877. PMID: 33061330; PMCID: PMC7533912.
27. Mills LG. The heart of intimate abuse: new interventions in child welfare, criminal justice, and health settings, Family violence series. Springer Publishing Company; 1998.
28. Findling MG, Bleich SN, Casey LS, Blendon RJ, Benson JM, Sayde JM, Miller C. Discrimination in the united states: experiences of latinos. Health Serv Res. 2019;54 Suppl 2(Suppl 2):1409–18.
29. Gómez CA, Kleinman DV, Pronk N, Wrenn Gordon GL, Ochiai E, Blakey C, Johnson A, Brewer KH. Addressing health equity and social determinants of health through healthy people 2030. J Public Health Manag Pract. 2021;27(Supplement 6):p S249–S257.
30. Vela MB, Erondu AI, Smith NA, Peek ME, Woodruff JN, Chin MH. Eliminating explicit and implicit biases in health care: evidence and research needs. Annu Rev Public Health. 2022;43:477–501. https://doi.org/10.1146/annurev-publhealth-052620-103528. Epub 2022 Jan 12. PMID: 35020445; PMCID: PMC9172268.
31. Data tool: demographics of the U.S. psychology workforce. American Psychological Association. 2022. https://www.apa.org/workforce/data-tools/demographics. Accessed 4 May 2024.
32. Koenig TL, Rinfrette ES, Lutz WA. Female caregivers' reflections on ethical decision-making: the intersection of domestic violence and elder care. Clin Soc Work J. 2006;34:361–72.
33. Calasanti T. Gender relations and applied research on aging. Gerontologist. 2010;50(6):720–34. https://doi.org/10.1093/geront/gnq085. Epub 2010 Oct 18.
34. Teaster P, Heisler G, Anetzberger G. Ethics and vulnerable elders. San Diego: Cognella; 2020. p. 219.
35. Code of Ethics. National Association of Social Workers. 2021. https://www.socialworkers.org/About/Ethics/Code-of-Ethics/Code-of-Ethics-English. Accessed 13Mar 2024.
36. Saghafi A, Bahramnezhad F, Poormollamirza A, Dadgari A, Navab E. Examining the ethical challenges in managing elder abuse: a systematic review. J Med Ethics Hist Med. 2019;12:7. PMID: 31346400; PMCID: PMC6642445.

Chapter 6
Unintentional Neglect

Lisa Gibbs, Pamela B. Teaster, and Marlena Orme

Introduction

Neglect is defined as withholding or failing to provide needed care to a vulnerable elder by a designated caregiver. Neglect can either be intentional or unintentional. Intentional neglect constitutes a deliberate act to refuse to provide the basics of shelter, nutrition, medical care and personal care. The abuser knows that they are withholding necessary care, and are capable, but are refusing to do so. Unintentional neglect is considered 'passive' neglect, where caregivers lack the ability, support, health literacy or resources to provide necessary care.

This chapter will focus on unintentional neglect of an older adult by her daughter.

Case Presentation

The physician, Dr. Myers, had only known Ms. M. for a brief period, as she had recently moved in with her daughter. Ms. M. had been living alone for the past 8 years in the home that she raised her family in. When Ms. M. suffered a fall one

L. Gibbs (✉)
Division of Geriatric Medicine and Gerontology, Department of Family Medicine, University of California, Irvine, CA, USA
e-mail: lgibbs@hs.uci.edu

P. B. Teaster
Center for Gerontology, Virginia Tech, Blacksburg, VA, USA

M. Orme
Burke Rehabilitation Center, White Plains, NY, USA

V. LoFaso, L. Rachmuth (eds.), *Elder Abuse and Neglect*,
https://doi.org/10.1007/978-3-031-97784-8_6

night, emergency services were called to help her get up. She was transported to the emergency room, and despite many areas of tenderness, no fractures were found. After it was clear that Ms. M needed more care, she moved in with her daughter. Ms. M. had been unable to maintain the upkeep of her house and her garden, which had previously given her much pleasure. She was also late in paying her bills, which was out of character for her.

During the initial visit, after hearing about initial comments from her daughter, Dr. Myers asked to speak with Ms. M. alone. After questioning her about her medical conditions and concerns, she was screened for cognitive impairment and falls risk. She screened positive for memory problems and for continued fall risk. In addition, she also asked Ms. M. about mood and purpose in life. Ms. M. answered that she enjoyed going to church frequently, social interactions and eating the food that she prefers. However, Ms. M. noted that she was unable to do these things as often as she would like to because she cannot drive and is reliant on her daughter for transportation. She notes that she is lonely and bored. The physician validated Ms. M.'s concerns by making a referral to the social worker in the office to offer resources.

Before the visit was over, Dr. Myers invited her daughter back into the exam room and explained her treatment plan. Her purpose was not only to explain next steps, but to include and educate her daughter in what a meaningful life meant to her mother.

During the second visit, 3 months later to follow up on the initial visit, Dr. Myers discovers that Ms. M. is as depressed and lonely as before. The social worker documented that he was unable to reach the patient or her daughter despite multiple attempts by telephone. Ms. M.'s daughter dismissed her mother's lack of socialization, community engagement, and loneliness, even after the physicians noted the effect on her overall health and wellbeing. Additional discussion revealed that they have never had a close relationship and that the daughter is a working single mom of two and feeling very overwhelmed. The social worker was asked to call or meet the daughter while she was in the office.

On the third visit, 2 months later, the nurse noted that she lost had lost 10 pounds in 4 months. Also, Dr. Myers noted that Ms. M.'s clothes were even more loose fitting than after her hospitalization and Sub Acute Rehabilitation stay, indicating additional weight loss. Whereas before rehabilitation, Ms. M. walked confidently with a walker, she now seemed to walked slowly and hesitantly. Her daughter noted that she had a fall in the bathroom and had bruises on her knees and legs. However, nothing seemed broken. Her daughter again presented as overwhelmed, tired and dismissive, and kept glancing at her watch and tapping her feet. When the doctor asked if she were worried about the time, she said she needed to pick up her daughter. Ms. M. looked away as if uncomfortable. The doctor senses the tension and asks her nurse to recheck Ms. M. blood pressure, excusing herself and her daughter.

Outside the room, Dr. Myers tells Ms. M.'s daughter that her mother is not doing well and that she is concerned about another fall. Her daughter insists that she is doing the best she can. When asks about what help she needs she says, 'We are fine. We don't need other people in our business. My mother wouldn't want that. The physician asks the daughter to wait in the waiting room and talks with Ms. M. about how she is doing. She feels that she is getting older and weaker, but that she does not want to be a burden. The physicians asks if the daughter has any issues with alcohol or substance use, and Ms. M. says no but that her daughter often drinks a lot of wine at night to relax.

Functionally, Ms. M. is declining. Her mobility is declining and needs hands-on assistance for transferring, toileting and bathing. Ms. M. cannot prepare her own meals, and her daughter relies on TV dinners for the family. This is very important as she is a diabetic and should adhere to a certain diet. She is able to use her telephone but has few remaining friends and family to call. She is alone during the day until her grandchildren and daughter arrive home at night.

Before they leave the office, the physicians has a very direct conversation with both her patient and daughter. She states that she is concerned about another fall, about weight look, about loneliness and that the daughter needs to look into resources, including adult daycare or having someone assist her mother during the day when she is alone. Dr. Myers notes that the daughter is the primary caregiver and that she is responsible, especially since her mother has some cognitive impairment. Ms. M. starts crying, saying she doesn't want to go to "a home". The physician schedules a follow-up in 2 weeks to check her weight.

At 2 weeks, the patient does not arrive for her appointment. At this point, the physician decides that, out of concern for her patient's wellbeing, she needs to report to Adult Protective Services.

Unintentional Neglect Overview

Healthcare providers are often the first to be aware that their patient may be experiencing neglect and for self-neglect. If patients have a designated caregiver, who clearly provides care for activities of daily living (ADLs) and instrumental activities of daily living (IADLs), and if these needs are not being met, then neglect, intentional or not, must be considered. When caring for older adults who are experiencing decline in their health or function, the important first step is to consider the cause. The care of frail older adults is often very complex, and a holistic approach is always best considering medical, social or psychological causes of decline. Patients should always be central to this conversation, with and without the caregiver present. If an older adult's quality of life is suffering, then consider what is needed and why this is missing. Identifying gaps in care can confirm that neglect is occurring and help formulate a plan going forward to address the neglect.

Unintentional neglect can be:

1. Physical Neglect—Lack of environmental basics, such as food, clothing, shelter, and personal care.

2. Medical Neglect—An individual's health is compromised by a caregiver's failure to seek timely medical care or follow a medical care plan, or by a refusal of needed medical service. [1]
3. Emotional Neglect—An individual's need for affection are consistently disregarded, ignored, invalidated, or unappreciated by a significant other. [2]
4. Self- Neglect—This describes "an adult's inability, due to physical or mental impairment or diminished capacity, to perform essential self-care tasks.", and includes "obtaining adequate food, water, clothing, shelter, personal hygiene, medical and mental health care, and safety precautions, and/or managing one's finances." [3]

The distinction between intentional and unintentional neglect can be challenging. Similar to other types of elder abuse, the intent behind the incident or circumstance is critical to understanding the behavior. If a caregiver has genuine intentions of caregiving and is receptive to recommendations for care, then unintentional neglect is likely. This includes ensuring that the vulnerable adult has ongoing medical care, has assistance for ADLs and IADLs, and social connection. However, if caregivers have an alternative agenda, such as refusing to assist because it takes effort or they have financial motives, then intentional neglect is likely. One of the more common scenarios for intentional neglect is when a child moves into the parent's home and does not contribute to the household expenses, or stable employment and lives off the older adult's income.

Financial causation is often at the root of both intentional and unintentional neglect. In the case of unintentional neglect, a caregiver or care recipient may lack the resources to hire the appropriate level of caregiving. The cost of both long-term insurance and paid caregiving is very expensive and a major concern of families caring for older adults. This often forces caregivers to make difficult choices, such as to whom and when to provide care and whether to retire early to meet the caregiving needs. While this may allow one to assume the hands on caregiving, families are left without the additional income they need for basic necessities of living. Difficult decisions may lead to feelings of resentment due to the loss of a career, or due to lack of support one has from other children or family members.

Social isolation is now considered an epidemic in the United States and a known risk factor for neglect. One study found that loneliness is as detrimental to health as smoking 15 cigarettes per day, leading to premature death [4] The emotional distress leads to depression and lack of motivation for self-care. Social connectedness is important for wellness, both psychological and physical. Even daily contact by meal delivery organizations ensures some human contact, thus improving quality of life.

Many older adults are susceptible to loneliness due to a variety of factors, including medical problems and cognitive decline. Medical conditions, such as arthritis, may be painful and increase the effort needed for mobility. Even daily activities such as driving, shopping, and walking distances may be challenging. Those with cognitive decline or dementia may be too self-conscious to socialize with friends who may notice memory problems. Incidentally, scammers and financial abuse criminals also target those at risk of loneliness and befriend them before gaining access to financial information. For those with dementia, the effects of social connectedness are believed to be critical for maintaining cognitive function.

For these reasons, access to community resources can be a lifeline for those experiencing loneliness. Community resources include home meal delivery, friendly visitor programs, or transportation to senior events, church related services, or relatives. Respite services may be available, which also provide needed breaks for the caregivers. In the United States, social service agencies are located in many counties or regions in each state.

Case Discussion

Consider what went right about this case. Dr. Myer established an open, caring, and collaborative interaction with Ms. M. through active listening and open-ended questions. She spoke with her alone and also followed an age friendly approach that provided essential valuable information and a holistic picture of Ms. M.'s situation. She understood that Ms. M. had just experienced a major life transition and was having difficulty in adjusting. Dr. Myer correctly included social worker assistance to broaden the understanding of Ms. M.'s life experience.

As the case unfolds, the importance of following up with a patient's plan and the value of a continuity relationship between healthcare clinicians and patients and caregivers becomes clearer. Dr Myer's careful questioning brought to light the overwhelming responsibilities the daughter had even before her mother moved in. The physician ensured that the social worker could communicate with Ms. M. and her daughter by having her meet them during the visit.

Subsequent follow-up visits clarified that initial attempts to provide Ms. M. and her daughter with resources have not improved her health and well- being, and in fact, Ms. M. is losing weight, feeling weaker, and has fallen again. Her daughter seems unable or unwilling to cope with the situation and is refusing additional assistance. She may also have an alcohol disuse disorder. The physician correctly spoke with the patient and her daughter alone to obtain a complete picture of the situation. The physician correctly realized that additional resources and education were needed to ensure that Ms. M. received the assistance she needed.

A healthcare professional only needs a suspicion of neglect or self-neglect to make a report. If the older adult has capacity, he or she can refuse to speak with the APS social worker. It is unclear at this point if the neglect is intentional and willful, or unintentional. The daughter is very clearly overwhelmed and using alcohol to cope. A whole lifetime of history exists between the mother and daughter, and it is unreasonable to expect a primary care physician to manage this situation without additional resources through the community.

In the case above, we do not have enough information to determine whether intentional or unintentional neglect is occurring. There is a concern for a strained relationship, knowing that the daughter and her mother have not been close until an acute situation has arisen. The daughter is struggling financially and a single parent for two children. We learn that there is a significant reliance on alcohol. Further assessment for the daughter should include questions about other substances, mental illness, and her other circumstances. Whether she has been the victim of trauma, such as intimate partner violence (IPV) may explain her reactions to stress. However, if she genuinely wants to care for her mother and incorporate her into her family, then continuing to approach her with understanding while ensuring her mother's safety, may lead to a successful outcome for both the caregiver and older adult. If the mother is deemed to be in an unsafe situation, or at high risk for complications such a traumatic injury or failure to thrive, then more aggressive interventions are necessary. In this case, Dr. Myers was so concerned that she called for APS involvement.

Even more important than understanding the capabilities, resources, and intent of the caregiver are the expressed preferences and needs of the patient. Understanding an older adult's wishes for where they prefer live and who cares for them as they continue to require more assistance is necessary for assuring independent decision making and personal dignity for the care recipient. In the primary care of older adults, these discussions should be considered early and over the course of the patient-clinician relationship, especially in the case of declining cognition and before a patient loses capacity. One useful tool for ensuring that these discussions take place is during the Medicare Annual Wellness Visit, where advance care planning is revisited every year.

Discussions about caregiving needs and functional decline often occur during stressful situations, such as an event requiring hospitalization and rehabilitation, diagnoses of dementia, or a change in living situations. The potential caregivers involved may need to change their lifestyle or alter their goals in life in order to provide adequate care. Many of these discussions ensue when families are in crisis and turn to healthcare professionals for help. In these situations, nonjudgmental and efficient communication is needed.

Active listening and asking open-ended questions will form the basis for communication. Creating a comfortable space and open rapport will result in trust and confidence among the parties. Beyond this, to understand an individual's understanding and motivation, using trauma-informed care and motivational interviewing skills will help move the conversation forward.

A history of trauma is unfortunately very prevalent in our society and is often uncovered in the dysfunction of families. The adoption of screening with ACEs is now a standard part of the care of children and abuse and violence as they are known to be intergenerational. Trauma-informed care was developed to help survivors of trauma with the principles of safety, trust, collaboration, empowerment, and cultural awareness [5, 9]. Motivational interviewing is evidence-based counseling that promote one own insight about resistance to change. There is empirical evidence that both together (Trauma Informed and Motivational Interviewing) helps clients who are self-neglecting to communicate with medical and legal professionals [5].

Examples of open-ended questions for potential caregivers:

- What is your understanding of the care your mother needs?
- We know that caregiving can be rewarding but difficult. How do you feel about being the primary caregiver for your mother?
- What type of assistance would be helpful for you to provide this care?
- How confident do you feel that you can provide this care on a scale from 1 to 10?

Examples of open-ended questions for vulnerable adults needing care:

- I am here to assist you-what type of assistance do you need right now?
- Who would you like to help you?
- Where would you like to live?
- What would make your daughter a successful caregiver? What difficulties do you thinks she would encounter
- Are you willing to receive help from the community such as meals on wheels? Would you consider participating in a senior center?
- If not, what would need to change so that we can get you more assistance?

Caregiver Stress and Its Consequences

When healthcare clinicians care for older adults requiring caregivers, attention must be extended to the caregiver as well. The health and wellbeing of caregivers directly affects the care of the care recipient. Increasing attention is being given to the role of caregiving as our population continues to age. Family members are often placed in the position of unpaid or informal caregiving. This situation may apply to children of older adults or partners and spouses of older adults or family members of dependent adults. Although many choose to be caregivers, others reluctantly agree to care for others in certain circumstances. Surely, caregiving can be very rewarding, especially if the carer and care recipient have a mutually beneficial relationship, and the caregiver has the support that they need. However, even in the best of circumstances, caregivers may feel stressed or burdened by the financial, physical, emotional, and mental stressors of caregiving.

Caregivers often ignore their own health and wellbeing needs. Many former caregivers present for their own care after their loved ones die, only to discover uncontrolled illnesses or missed opportunities for preventive measures. If caregivers are forced to give up their paid employment, there may be a financial burden as well. Having concurrent parental responsibilities raises the risk of caregiver burden. One review of several articles on determinant of caregiving burden found that the extent of the burden correlated with the duration of care and the level of caregiving needed per day [6].

Asking caregivers how they are doing is always greatly appreciated. Further asking what support and assistance they need can be enlightening and can lead to referrals for community services and counseling. Objective measures of caregiver burden through validated scales also provides baseline information that can be tracked over time.

Assessment of the Older Adult

Geriatric medicine is known for a comprehensive assessment, including medical conditions, medications, mental health, mobility, function and social support. Depending on individual medical offices, this information can be gathered by a team, by a single clinician in a single setting, or over time as in a continuity of care relationship.

- *It is necessary to communicate with the patient in their primary language.* Use an interpreter service and not a family member, even if the patient and caregiver insist. Some information might be interpreted differently, left out or filtered when using a family member or friend to interpret your medical and clinical interactions.
- *Make it part of your practice to meet with the patient alone for a portion of time during your visit.* However, including the caregiver also provides insight and collateral information during the interaction. During the patient's visit, the caregiver is also being assessed. Caregivers often play a critical role in the patient's care and should be Included as care partners.
- *Observe for caregiver and patient interactions.* How do they communicate? Does your patient exhibit fear or hesitancy or lack of confidence to speak?
- *Establish who has caregiving role(s) and what assistance is provided.* Assess whether this matches your patient's needs.

  When working with older adults, providers often assume that the caregiver will take on certain roles and responsibility without formally asking or assessing if they can meet the patient's needs. Providers need to be clear on what they are asking the caregivers to do. Never assume the caregiver is willing and able to perform a necessary task.

- *Perform physical observations/exam.*

  Is your patient well appearing? Observation includes grooming, cleanliness, clipped nails, and appropriate clothing. Are they comfortable or in pain or anxious? How did they arrive? Did they drive (and should they be driving?)or were they accompanied? Did they have the durable medical equipment they require? This may include glasses, hearing aids, rolling walker or canes.

- *Assess function to inform what assistance and level of care your patient needs.*

  Ask how your patient actively participates in life? How do they function in the world, and do they get their basic needs met? Make it a point to assess each of the Activities of Daily living and Independent Activities of Daily living. What do they need help with?

  Activities of Daily Living are the basic activities needed for daily life and include transferring, dressing, toileting, and eating.

IADLs require a higher level of functioning and interfacing with our community. IADLs include activities such as managing finances, medications, preparing meals, and shopping for groceries.

Age-Friendly Care

Many clinicians caring for older adults use a set of evidence-based practices to ensure a holistic approach to patient care. Many health systems are now designated as Age Friendly, which align with what matters to older adults and their caregivers and promotes quality of care. This includes the '5 M's, which stand for Mentation, Medications, Mobility, what Matters Most, and Multicomplexity [5]. Each of these is covered below with respect to the prevention and assessment for neglect or self-neglect.

Mentation

This M includes screening and addressing dementia, depression and delirium. All of this impact the risk for neglect and self-neglect. Dementia is a known risk for elder abuse. Studies show that up to 50% of demented patients experience some form of abuse [7]. The presence of dementia also increases the responsibilities for the caregiver, depending on whether the cognitive deficits are mild, moderate, or advanced. Screening for cognitive decline annually is an important assessment to understand how memory may affect new functional deficits. Dementia related behaviors, which may include physical violence, or fear of basic activities significantly increase the stress of caregiving and may cause verbal or physical aggression in addition to a hands-off approach to caregiving which may lead to neglect.

In addition, as patients with dementia live with the disease, their capacity is affected. Initially, it will affect complex tasks such as financial management but later will affect more basic decisions.

Caregivers need education to understand that capacity must be expressly evaluated and cannot be assumed because someone has mild or moderate dementia. Sometimes caregivers may take too much control of their life and environment without respecting autonomy. Or the caregiver might allow too much independence and jeopardize the patient's safety, not fully realizing the limitation for decision making. Having this conversation with the caregiver and patient over time is part of primary care practice for dementia.

Depression also has risks for neglect and self-neglect. Depression is associated with loneliness, functional decline and the ability to care for oneself. It affects the caregiver's role and relationship with the vulnerable adults. Vulnerable adults may lack the energy to help themselves and refuse assistance from caregivers.

Medications

Medication use or lack of use is often the major clue to the presence of neglect and self-neglect. Certainly, most chronic diseases such as diabetes, hypertension, and movement disorders require ongoing medications. If the chronic disease management isn't effective, consider that the caregiver may not be administering the patient's medication appropriately. Sometimes caregivers do not realize that patients are not capable of managing their own medications. Dementia, depression and delirium are common reasons for medication mismanagement.

- Are the patient's medications appropriate? If not, is the medication filled on schedule? Consider a pain medication contract and urine testing for the medication.

Mobility

Mobility-related issues are important for preventing immobility and falls. Falls in frail older adults are often the one event that affects independence and mortality [8]. Attention to safely maintaining mobility is a key responsibility for a caregiver. Medical professionals should conduct an evidence-based gait and balance assessment to determine whether patients present a fall risk. Equipment such as canes, walkers, rollators and wheelchairs may be needed. When a more in-depth assessment is needed, a referral to physical therapy is warranted. The caregiver should then follow recommendations and ensure patient adherence to mobility aids. If a patient is bedbound, or needs maximum assistance for mobility, the caregiver should ensure proper skin care to prevent pressure injuries. If a patient is bedbound an assessment for a pressurized air mattress should be completed along with education for turning patients on a routine basis. If caregivers ignore these recommendations, putting the patient at risk for falls and pressure injury, then neglect should be considered.

Matters Most

As illustrated above in the case study, it is crucial to keep the patient's wishes and goals in the foreground. If the patient has capacity to make decisions then they should be respected even if the care team does not agree with them. The right to personal autonomy can sometimes leave clinicians in an uncomfortable position, and attempts to keep the patient safe may be thwarted. Ongoing follow-up, involving community agencies and keeping lines of communication open are helpful strategies to keep the older adult safe.

Multicomplexity

The more burden of disease an older adult has, the more vulnerable and dependent they are for care. This puts them at risk for abuse and neglect. More physical needs place a higher burden of care on the older adults caregiver. In many cases the caregivers are not able to meet those needs and neglect occurs. When older adults have significant medical and psychiatric problems polypharmacy, multiple medical providers, and disjointed care can result. If the older adult does not have a primary care physician they see regularly, subtle changes in their health status that might indicate neglect can be easily overlooked.

Clinicians with and without social work support should take the time to research and be familiar with community based services and how they might be helpful to your practice. Building a list of resources available for social determinates of health needs will be helpful, and information flyers may be given to patients and caregiver.

Social Work Perspective

Knowing your patient's culture, religion, lifestyle, and background are important for honest and open communication and allows the healthcare professional to know 'what matters most' to their patients. Knowing one's own biases is important to practice nonjudgmental medical care. For instance, what are your thoughts towards older adults, and how might this influence your perception of the unintentional neglect discussed above? In many cases of neglect, there is a tendency to sympathize with caregivers, even in the face of clear malintent, due to personal experiences caregiving stress. Does your culture assume that children will step up and take care of their parents when they get older? Would a caregiver's or care recipient's race, culture or sexual orientation or gender expression play a role in your perception? Was there trauma in the past, such as a history of domestic violence, and would that change your view of the caregiver or patient?

In fact, ageism itself is a common bias and results in discrimination and stereotyping. Ageism affects healthcare decisions with beliefs that older people can't recover, patients with dementia can't make decisions, or 'old people die'. Expectations for caregivers may be affected by ageist attitudes towards the care recipients. As with all good geriatric care, obtaining an in-depth social history, including a values history, and approaching the client without bias or ageist attitudes will yield the best results for older adult patients.

Health professionals have a professional mandate to advocate and protect our older adults because they have the access to patients and caregivers and the knowledge and skills to provide the care they need. By understanding neglect, whether intentional or unintentional and how to respond, we can make the difference for a healthier and happier lives for our patients.

The education that you provide is an essential aspect of your interventions. Ask yourself why a meeting might be necessary and set a clear agenda. Set up a formal meeting or intentional conversation with the patient and or caregiver. Avoid making assumptions of their knowledge and making a fleeting comment in a short interaction. This is especially important when providing education about an act or lack of action that could be considered neglect. This serves a double purpose of highlighting the importance of the issue being discussed as well as educating the patient and caregiver in a practical way that could reduce or eliminate neglect. Making this a strategic intervention sends the message that what we are about to discuss is important.

Preparation will help you organize your thoughts, your concerns and your goals for the educational session. Begin by making sure the setting is quiet and that you are at eye level with the people with whom you are talking. This helps to build rapport and is non threating. Then, thank the patient and or caregiver for taking the time to meet with you.

Start by asking the patient their perception of their current situation. This will give the clinician information about whether the patient has insight into the reality of their situation.

Use simple terms to explain or educate. Incorporate different modalities in your education, whether that is handouts or visuals. How does this person learn? Are they visual? Do they need written material? Ask and provide assistance if necessary. Encourage attendees to take notes and provide any relevant educational information or handouts.

After you have provided the appropriate education, use the teach-back method. Ask the patient or caregiver to retell the key information in their own words. Look for gaps and provide the missing information as needed.

Be available post-meeting to answer questions the patient or caregiver might have thought of post-education. Provide them with a way to contact you if needed. This might also be difficult depending on your place of employment and time constraints.

Take the time to provide education in a culturally responsive and comprehensive way. As previously stated, communicate and use materials in the person's primary language, both written and verbal. What did the patient or caregiver teach you? What have you learned about the gaps in the patient's needs and what are the barriers to filling them? What did you learn about the patient and caregiver during the meeting, and does this information change your interventions?

Emotional and Mental Health Interventions

Are there any psychological and mental health concerns that are barriers to meeting the needs of a patient that should be addressed? Does the patient's mental health influence their openness to care and services? Have they lost interest in their own care and wellbeing? Any patient mental health concerns should be addressed.

Does the caregiver need emotional support and or mental health services? Is there any substance abuse that needs to be addressed? If a caregiver is suffering from depression or caregiver burnout, you can imagine they might have a hard time sleeping, and or concentrating making it challenging for them to take care of others.

This might be perceived as and contributing to the unintentional neglect. The caregiver may have good intentions but faling short because they and need professional mental health intervention themselves. Be an advocate for your patient and their caregiver. If you made the referral, follow up with the agency as well as your patient/caregiver to ensure services have been assessed.

Behaviors and mental health do not change overnight. They take time and effort on behalf of the patient and the caregiver. Assess the intention of treatment and intervention and level of engagement of the patient and caregiver. Encourage caregivers to get assistance from other family, friends, or community resources. Problem solve and help the caregiver identify options to accept help and offload some of the caregiver responsibilities. The caregiver might consider trying to access home care services or respite care from any agency or other support system.

Adult Protective Service Referral

Determine if and when to make a referral to an Adult Protective Service agency. If the risk is imminent and high for severe harm or death, it is important to make the referral. Also consider making the referral if follow through has not occurred related to all previously suggested interventions. Regardless of whether the mistreatment is intentional or unintentional, the patient is still at risk for harm and may have little to no chance for recovery.

Not all states have mandated reporting laws and regulations. Know your state's requirements. Even if you are not a mandated reporter, you might feel uncomfortable and uncertain about what to do next. Determine your ethical obligations to protect a vulnerable adult who cannot meet their own needs. Making an APS referral can be daunting and stressful, so consider making the call with a supervisor or trusted colleague. Remember, if you are concerned about someone, your role is to bring the case to APS to evaluate, not to determine if there is mistreatment happening.

Ethical Dilemmas: What if no neglect is found? What if the patient refuses help? What will happen to your patient/caregiver relationship and rapport? Prior to making a referral, ask yourself what interventions APS can provide that you, a social worker on staff or community case manager, cannot provide.

Be aware of your own basis for action and how it might influence your assessment and interventions. Often, in such cases as the one presented, people have to make difficult choices and must choose the best choice among bad choices. Being a non-judgemental partner and advocate can make a significant difference in the lives of older adults and their families.

Key Points

- Neglect can be intentional or unintentional. Determining the intent of the caregiver is crucial to distinguishing these two forms of mistreatment.
- Social isolation, cognitive impairment, and high burden of care are risk factors for neglect.

- Indicators to elder neglect include decline in previously stable medical conditions, weight loss, dehydration, changes in personal care and hygeine, lack of assistive devices, and depression.
- Interviewing victims of neglect should occur in a safe, quiet environment in the absence of the alleged perpetrator.
- In cases of neglect, assessing caregiver burden and stress is crucial. Interventions to reduce stress and support caregivers can improve their ability to provide care to the older adult.
- Societal ageist attitudes and cultural biases can be barriers to effectively evaluating and intervening in cases of neglect.
- Healthcare professionals have a unique opportunity to detect and intervene in cases of neglect. Using a multidisciplinary team approach is the most effective approach to assessing a neglectful situation.
- Careful documentation of all physical findings, observations, and interactions is imperative.

References

1. Stirling J. Understanding medical neglect: when needed care is delayed or refused. J Child Adolesc Trauma. 2019;13(3):271–6.
2. Ludwig S, Rostain A Chapter 10: Family function and dysfunction.In: Developmental-behavioral pediatrics. 4th ed., pp. 103–118. https://doi.org/10.1016/B978-1-4160-3370-7.00010-9. https://www.sciencedirect.com/science/book/9781416033707
3. Graham J. 'They Treat Me Like I'm Old and Stupid': seniors decry health providers' age bias. Kaiser Health News, October 20, 2021.
4. Holt-Lunstad J, Robles TF, Sbarra DA. Advancing social connection as a public health priority in the United States. Am Psychol. 2017;72(6):517–30.
5. Hopper EK, Bassuk EL, Oliver J. Shelter from the storm: trauma-informed care in homelessness services settings. Open Health Serv Policy J. 2010;3:80–100.
6. Lindt N, Berkel J, Mulder BC. Determinants of overburdening among informal carers: a systematic review. BMC Geriatr. 2020;20:304. https://doi.org/10.1186/s12877-020-01708-3.
7. Wiglesworth A, Mosqueda L, Mulnard R, Liao S, Gibbs L, Fitzgerald W. Screening for abuse and neglect of people with dementia. J Am Geriatr Soc. 2010;58(3):493–500. https://doi.org/10.1111/j.1532-5415.2010.02737.x.
8. Tom SE, Adachi JD, Anderson FA Jr, Boonen S, Chapurlat RD, Compston JE, Cooper C, Gehlbach SH, Greenspan SL, Hooven FH, Nieves JW, Pfeilschifter J, Roux C, Silverman S, Wyman A, LaCroix AZ, GLOW Investigators. Frailty and fracture, disability, and falls: a multiple country study from the global longitudinal study of osteoporosis in women. J Am Geriatr Soc. 2013;61(3):327–34. https://doi.org/10.1111/jgs.12146. Epub 2013 Jan 25. PMID: 23351064; PMCID: PMC3602412.
9. Ellis E, Martino S, Simiola V, Bellamy C, O'Connell M, Cook JM. Training male sexual abuse survivors as peer leaders to deliver motivational interviewing and trauma-informed affirmative care. J Child Sex Abus. 2023;32(4):494–512. https://doi.org/10.1080/10538712.2023.2203691.

Suggested Reading

NCEA: https://ncea.acl.gov/elder-abuse#gsc.tab=0

Chapter 7
Intentional Neglect

Veronica LoFaso and Page Ulrey

Introduction

Neglect is defined as the failure of a responsible caregiver to meet the medical, social and/or psychological needs of an older adult resulting in risk of harm, actual harm, or death. Older adult victims of neglect are among the most vulnerable cohort, often unable or unwilling, because of shame or fear, to report the neglect to authorities. Perpetrators of neglect can be family members, paid or unpaid caregivers, or institutions [1]. Neglect can be either unintentional, as discussed in the previous chapter or intentional, perpetrated with the knowing and willing intent to inflict harm. Intentional neglect, the subject of this chapter, can rise to the level of criminality with the degree of harm required dependent on state law.

The high incidence of elder abuse and neglect is generally accepted, although recognized to be underreported [2]. Ascertaining the exact prevalence of elder neglect, intentional or unintentional, is difficult because of study designs and discrepancies in the definitions used in studies. To date the literature estimates that elder neglect accounts for 11.6% of all elder abuse cases, ranking third after psychological and financial abuse [3]. The following scenario describes a case of intentional criminal neglect, which rose to the level of criminal, which was referred to the district attorney's office by law enforcement after responding to a 911 call.

V. LoFaso (Retired) (✉)
Division of Geriatrics and Palliative Medicine, Weill Cornell Medicine, New York, NY, USA
e-mail: Vel2001@med.cornell.edu

P. Ulrey
Elder Abuse Unit, King County Prosecuting Attorney's Office, Seattle, WA, USA

V. LoFaso, L. Rachmuth (eds.), *Elder Abuse and Neglect*,
https://doi.org/10.1007/978-3-031-97784-8_7

Case Presentation

Ms S. was an 88-year-old woman who had been living with her adult son for the past 3 years. She was a strong-willed woman who had previously lived by herself and valued her independence. Her son had noticed mild cognitive changes as long as 5 years ago but felt that in the last few years she had significantly declined and needed more oversight. He responded by moving her to a house on the west coast which they then shared until the time of her death. She died in her bed at home and her son called 911 to report her death. Upon arriving, Emergency Medical Services (EMS) personnel walked into Ms S.' room, pronounced her dead, and, following protocol, called law enforcement. EMS did not note any concerns about the condition of her body in their report. Law enforcement arrived and immediately noticed a terrible odor in the home. They pulled back the covers and found Ms S.to be emaciated with multiple severe pressure ulcers, bruises and showing signs of extremely poor hygiene. Though her lower body was smeared with feces, her diaper and sheets were clean. She had blood underneath her overgrown fingernails. A homicide detective was assigned to the case and immediately started an investigation. The detective requested that the medical examiner's office come to the scene and called the prosecutor's office to consult with them on how to proceed. The autopsy revealed that Ms S. had suffered from severe malnutrition, dehydration, multiple advanced and infected pressure ulcers and bruises. Additional information gathered later in the investigation revealed that Ms S. had been diagnosed with dementia, and that her son was a single, unemployed computer engineer who lived off her retirement benefits. As Ms S. declined, he had turned down offers of in-home care and long-term care for his mother. After the investigation was concluded, the prosecutor's office filed the charge of Manslaughter in the First Degree against Ms S's son.

Victim's Medical History

- Hypothyroidism
- Hypertension
- Mild congestive heart failure
- Aortic stenosis
- Carotid stenosis
- Urinary incontinence
- Osteoporosis
- Hearing loss
- Vision impairment/cataracts
- Depression
- Cognitive impairment was reported in medical charts although no formal testing performed

Surgical History

- (S/P) bilateral total hip replacement
- S/P shoulder surgery bilaterally

Medications
- Levothyroxine 0.05 mg daily for hypothyroidism
- Alendronate 150 mg weekly for osteoporosis
- Losartan 25 mg daily for high blood pressure
- Furosemide 20 mg daily for fluid retention

Laboratory Data
- Toxicology screen negative

Autopsy Report
Pertinent findings:

- Height 4′11"
- Weight 72 pounds
- Evidence of emaciation and dehydration
- Perineum covered in feces
- Bilateral incipient heel ulcers
- Toenails thickened, long and irregular
- Fingernails long and dirty
- Scars from previous shoulder and hip surgeries
- Osteopenia
- Emphysematous changes
- Arterionephrosclerosis
- Cardiac atherosclerosis
- Cerebral cortex: gyral atrophy and scattered plaques, tangles and focal gliosis especially in hippocampus.
- 14 areas of ulceration: upper extremities, torso, scapular region, sacrum, hip, extremities, feet. Several of the pressure ulcers were necrotic and extended to bone with evidence of osteomyelitis
- Multiple bruises over extremities bilaterally in various stages of healing

Intentional Neglect Overview

Recognition of elder abuse and neglect, as a criminal act and therefore prosecutable, came to the fore in the 1990s. Prior to that, most cases of abuse and neglect were evaluated by Adult Protective Services (APS) or other community agencies and rarely referred to law enforcement. If cases were filed, they were brought to civil court [4]. Over the last two decades, with increasing knowledge and awareness, the frequency of criminal prosecutions of elder abuse and neglect has increased. These cases, however, remain a challenge for the criminal justice system.

The definition of criminal neglect differs from state to state. Neglect, in general, becomes criminal when the facts of a case rise to the level of a crime in the jurisdiction in which it occurred. In most states, criminal neglect statutes contain the following elements:

- the defendant has a duty of care to the victim
- the defendant acts with criminal negligence, recklessness, or intent
- the defendant's failure to provide care causes death, harm, or an imminent risk of harm to the victim
- the victim is dependent on the defendant for the basic necessities of life [5].

The previous chapter described a case of neglect that does not rise to the level of a crime; this case presents an instance of criminal neglect. Such neglect can include withholding life-sustaining medications and/or medical care, denying the older adult assistive devices such as hearing aids, dentures, glasses and canes or walkers. In addition, withholding access to adequate food and hydration, heating or air conditioning and proper hygiene are also hallmarks of elder criminal neglect. The determinative factor for criminal neglect is that the withholding of one of these needs causes the dependent person harm, imminent risk of harm, or death. It must also demonstrate the requisite intent, which varies by state. Though neglect most often occurs with older adults that lack capacity, it can also occur if an older adult with capacity is so functionally impaired they cannot seek help. An abusive caregiver may be isolating the patient from family and community, thus cutting off critical access to care, subsequently causing harm. A case of elder neglect can rise to the level of a criminality and yet still not be appropriate for prosecution. A common example of this is when the caregiver is the adult child of the victim and lacks the basic skills to provide care to the parent, perhaps because of a developmental disability or mental illness.

Elder abuse prosecutors, when making decisions to file charges, increasingly look for the presence of a financial motive on the part of the caregiver to neglect the elder. Health care providers need to remain cognizant of the fact that when confronted with concerning cases of neglect, they should report those cases to the authorities so that an investigation can be conducted and proper steps taken. Health care providers are also usually required by their state mandatory reporting laws to report neglect to authorities. Sometimes health care providers presume that the caregiver is well-intentioned and fail to report a case of neglect, resulting in the elder's unnecessary suffering and/or death [6, 7].

Identifying neglect that may rise to the level of criminality is challenging for health care providers. When an older adult presents to a health care facility with bruising or a suspicious fracture, an astute clinician has a tangible clue to possible elder abuse. Elder neglect is more subtle. Victims can suffer in silence for years before the mistreatment is uncovered. The reasons for this are not surprising. The changes of aging, including weight loss, diminishing functional status, dehydration, and pressure ulcers, can mimic neglect [8, 9]. Determining what is normal aging and what is neglect requires careful review of previous records and input from many sources. Ageism on the part of the health care system and society at large may result in care providers' expecting their older adult patients to be frail, eat less, be less hydrated and present as depressed. Sadly, all these findings, which may too easily be dismissed, may be signs of serious neglect. Many older adults will not report their neglectful caregiver for fear of retaliation, concern about a loved one having to engage with the criminal justice system, or most commonly, fear of being forced to move to a long-term care facility. Even post-mortem exams by medical examiners sometimes mischaracterize disturbing physical findings consistent with neglect as signs of normal aging [8]. This may be the result of lack of experience and training, insufficient history from facilities or medical personnel, or simply ageist assumptions.

When to Consider Criminality

Physicians are concerned with supporting, educating and intervening in whatever way possible to improve difficult situations; they are seldom focused on the legal consequences of neglect by caregivers. Some cases of neglect, however, are so egregious that the perpetrators must be held accountable. Serious cases of criminal neglect can and should be prosecuted. Why then is prosecution so challenging?

Only recently have elder abuse, neglect, and exploitation begun to be recognized as potentially criminal by the legal system [4]. In order to prove criminal neglect, most states require that the roughly same elements be proved. One such element that the state must prove is that the defendant had actually assumed the role of the victim's caregiver. But what legally defines a caregiver? Is it the responsibility of the adult child to care for the impaired parent? No states in the U.S. impose any duty of care of aging parents by their adult children. In general, however, if an adult child, or any other adult, assumes responsibility to become the caregiver for the dependent older adult, they are committing to providing the basic necessities of life for that individual. They then can be subject to prosecution if they subsequently fail to provide care to the dependent person, resulting in death or serious harm, or putting the dependent person in imminent risk of death or serious harm.

Another element that must typically be proved in prosecuting criminal neglect is intent. The level of intent required varies by state. In many states, the prosecution must show that the caregiver acted with recklessness or criminal negligence [10]. In Washington State, for example, the intent requirement, called Criminal Mistreatment, is criminal negligence. It is defined as "when (a person) fails to be aware of a substantial risk that (a wrongful act) may occur and this failure constitutes a gross deviation from the standard of care that a reasonable person would exercise in the same situation" (WPIC 10.04) Finally, it must typically be proven that the risk of harm, harm, or death the victim sustained was a result of the neglect and not a result of aging or underlying disease.

Most state neglect laws are written to preclude the prosecution of a caregiver who lacks the intellectual capacity or means to carry out needed care. Clearly, it is not for us as health care providers to make these determinations. What health care providers can and should do when concerned about the care their patient is receiving is thoroughly document the patient's statements and those of the caregiver (including their willingness to act as the designated caregiver), document any wounds or pressure sores and signs and symptoms of neglect, obtain a thorough social history and assess the patient's cognitive status. If after a thorough assessment there is concern for the patient's safety and well-being then reporting the case to Adult Protective Services and/or the police, depending on your state's mandatory reporting requirements is indicated. Even if in doubt it is best to report.

Considerations for Health Care Clinicians

Experienced social workers and Adult Protective Services workers are key collaborators in collecting the pertinent facts of a case needed by prosecutors to make an ethical and informed decision about criminality. If the clinician has concerns that the neglect may reach the level of criminality, the following aspects of the case should be fleshed out and documented (Table 7.1).

Table 7.1 Common findings at autopsy in cases of neglect

Condition leading to harm/death	Physical Findings	Cause
Dehydration	Sunken eyes, skin tenting, elevated serum sodium, renal impairment [11]	Withholding fluids
Malnutrition	Cachexia (BMI < 20), Low albumin or pre-albumin, low cholesterol, low vitamin levels	Lack of proper nutrition
Pressure ulcers	Multiple ulcers, advanced stage, untreated, infected	Improper positioning, lack of turning, improper mattress, poor nutrition and hydration, untreated or improperly treated wounds
Medication mismanagement	Absence or low levels of prescribed medications, i.e. thyroid replacement, blood thinners, seizure meds etc.	Medications not purchased or administered
Poor hygiene/skin rashes	Fungal infections, diaper rash, soiled diapers/bedclothes, poor nail care, poor dentition	Lack of assistance in bathing and grooming
Infection/sepsis	Cellulitis, fungal infections, osteomyelitis, pneumonia	Untreated wounds, impaired immunity, malnutrition
Hypo/hyperthermia	Above 104 °F Body temperature <95 °F or.	Lack of heat or AC

Physical Findings

Parsing out normal aging from neglect requires a rigorous review of medical data and historical information. Dehydration, for example, which is often seen in older adults, can be related to many causes [12]. The most often causes include decreased thirst sensation, certain medications (i.e. diuretics), chronic or acute illness (i.e. diarrhea or vomiting) or failure of the older kidney to concentrate urine [13]. Hypernatremia (elevated sodium levels greater than 145 mmol/L) is a potentially life-threatening result [14]. One study found a 33% mortality rate when serum levels in a geriatric population rose above 151. Another study found 50% of patients hospitalized with dehydration died within a year. The mortality rate was 74% for those with serum sodium levels above 154 [15, 16] Medical examiners describe severe dehydration as a key finding in forensic cases. Collins et al. describe eight cases of elder neglect reviewed by the ME, three of which were ascribed to severe dehydration. Post-mortem vitreous sodium levels were 164 and BUN levels between 76–310 mg/dL [17].

Criminally negligent caregivers may withhold fluids to overtly harm the victim and hasten death, to reduce the need for providing personal hygiene and changing of bedclothing, or simply because they choose to be inattentive to the victim's needs. Whatever the motive, older adults' lack of physiologic reserve can make dehydration a significant contributor to morbidity or death [18].

Malnutrition is another common finding in criminal neglect cases that is also often found in the geriatric population at large. Older adults often have reduced sensations of taste and smell, making food less palatable. They may have dental or gastrointestinal or swallowing disorders that discourage desire for food. They may be taking medications that are affecting their appetite. End-stage dementia can cause the release of TNF (Tumor Necrosis Factor) that can contribute to weight loss. Malignancy can result in weight loss as can endocrine disorders, such as hyperthyroid or uncontrolled diabetes, and COPD.

The above conditions can all contribute to weight loss and can be explained. In the absence of a plausible explanation, however, neglect rises in the differential diagnosis of weight loss. Clinicians become concerned when there is a change in weight greater than 10–15% of baseline body weight in a 6–12-month period. A BMI less than 21 kg/m or a triceps skinfold and mid-arm circumference less than 80% of normal are considered highly abnormal [18, 19] Medical examiners report malnutrition among the most telling factors in determining abuse. In a large retrospective study over 10 years, 36.4% of post-mortem neglect cases exhibited severe malnutrition (BMI <17.5 Kg/m^2) and 40.9% were underweight (BMI 17.5–20 kg/m^2). Collins reports that of the eight neglect cases brought to medical examiner review, seven were cachectic [17].

Laboratory findings can be helpful in documenting malnutrition. Low levels of certain proteins manufactured in the liver such as albumin, pre-albumin, and transferrin may be noted. Unusually low cholesterol levels and low levels of vitamins and trace elements such as Vitamin D, Vitamin B, folate, thiamine, pyridoxine and riboflavin can be clues as well.

Pressure ulcers (PU), dehydration, and malnutrition are frequently considered the three hallmarks of criminal neglect. Yet the incidence of PU is quite common, having been reported as high as 0.4–38% in acute care settings, 2.2–23.9% in LTC facilities and 0–17% in home care [20]. PU are in general an indicator of overall poor health status and overall poor prognosis and are found frequently in patients with diabetes, COPD, and end-stage dementia. PU lead to extended hospital stays, decrease in function and increased morbidity and mortality.

Although there are many postulated strategies to prevent pressure ulcers, they can occur even with good care. There are reports of pressure ulcers developing within hours during prolonged surgical procedures [20]. The concern for neglect is raised in the following situations:

1. Multiple pressure ulcers -particularly in areas that can be easily protected by repositioning
2. Ulcers in advanced stages (National Pressure Injury Advisory Panel stage 3 or 4)
3. Evidence of infected ulcers (cellulitis/osteomyelitis)
4. Untreated ulcers
5. Absence of proper mattress/pressure reducing devices
6. Obvious poor hygiene/skin rashes
7. Lack of documentation and consultation with medical or nursing professionals

Cognitive Impairment

Elderly patients often exhibit physical and/or cognitive impairments that result in their need for the assistance of a caregiver. A caregiver who is suspected of committing neglect may explain their actions by claiming that they were merely complying with the victim's wishes. In all cases of potential neglect, it is, therefore, crucial to know the victim's capacity to make decisions about their care. If the older adult truly is refusing services with full knowledge of their decision and freedom to make it, and has capacity to decline those services, then there is no culpability on the part of the caregiver. An investigators's determination of the basis of the older adult's decision making can be complex and, unfortunately, it is often made retrospectively after the victim is deceased, based on record review alone. If the patient's cognitive status is in question, cognitive capacity must be determined by a health care professional with training and experience in conducting evaluations of people with dementia. Sometimes an older adult with capacity will refuse medical or home care, as they have every right to do. They may lose the capacity to decide on their care if their cognitive condition declines and as dementia or delirium worsens. At that point the caregiver must make reasonable decisions about proper care that are consistent with the older adult's wishes but also provide pain control and dignity.

Access to Medical Care

Neglectful caregivers commonly prevent the older adult from accessing medical care-either in or out of the home. Often it is determined, retrospectively, that office visits were not attended and medical advice was not heeded by the caregiver. It is helpful for investigators to know the history of the victim's relationship with the health care system. Was there, for example, an established pattern of accessing health care in the past that is different now that this caregiver is in control? To avoid recognition of any pattern of neglect or abuse abusers will often move the victim's health care from one provider to another or use emergency room visits. Not infrequently, abusers will simply abandon the victim in the emergency room. Any unexplained change in a patient's chronic illness management should trigger an investigation as to why there is a change. There are many possible options, but consideration should be given to possible neglect. Were medications given appropriately? Was pain controlled? Were infections treated? Was proper hygiene maintained? Signs of dehydration, malnutrition or uncared for pressure ulcers should raise a red flag as should improper bedding and mattresses and lack of assistive devices. Each of these questions helps to assess the level of engagement and oversight of the caregiver and the risk the patient faces.

Condition of the Victim's Physical Environment

The condition of the victim's environment can give insight into their overall care. Did they have heat or air conditioning? Was the room clean? Were bedclothes maintained? Were there insects or vermin? Did they have access to a bathroom? Did they have access to a telephone? Personal response system? Television? Perhaps most importantly, did the victim's living space seem very different from that of the caregiver's, suggesting a lack of concern for the older adult and lack of prioritization of their needs over the caregiver's. In many cases the victim is relegated to a small, uncomfortable room while the caregiver lives in a much larger, more comfortable space.

Potential Motives

Sometimes a neglectful family caregiver will avoid spending the older adult's money on needed care so they can protect their inheritance. Or, more commonly, they will keep the older adult in the home to avoid the older adult's income stream from being diverted to a care facility or in-home caregivers. When considering criminal neglect, consideration should be given to the possibility of the caregiver financially benefitting from the death of the older adult or from keeping the older adult in the home rather than having to pay for a long-term care facility or in-home care.

Relationship Between Perpetrator and Victim

Characterizing the nature of the relationship between the perpetrator and the victim is a critical piece of the larger puzzle that investigator's must condsider. Was there long-standing enmeshment between the two? Animosity? Dependency? Was this a family where violence was ongoing for years? Was there perceived caregiver stress? Often the perpetrator suffers from mental illness or substance abuse. Adult children neglecters are frequently unemployed, have unsuccessful work histories and live off the income of their parent. They may also have addictions, such as gambling, shopping, or drugs, that drive their need to avoid the expense of needed home care workers or nursing home placement for the victim.

Contribution of Collateral Information

When a health care worker becomes concerned about a case of potential criminal neglect it is helpful to know if there is a history of dysfunction in the family. A social worker can assist in obtaining important collateral information from family and friends and community agencies. Have neighbors reported hearing screaming or fighting? Can other family members help establish a motive? Has there been physical abuse in the past requiring police reports? Has Adult Protective Services (APS) been called in in the past for reports of abuse or neglect? Has there ever been an order of protection? This information can often fill in the blanks in cases where neglect is in question.

Social Isolation

Social isolation is a common thread in cases of adult neglect especially those that rise to the level of being criminal. The victim is typically entirely dependent on the neglecting caregiver and has few if any other social contacts. Health care providers of vulnerable older patients need to ask them about their social contacts and support, document the patient's answers, and engage a social worker and/or report to APS when there is a concern that a patient is socially isolated and their caregiver lacks the ability to or is not committed to providing them with the care they need.

Assessing Possibility of Intentional Neglect (Fig. 7.1).

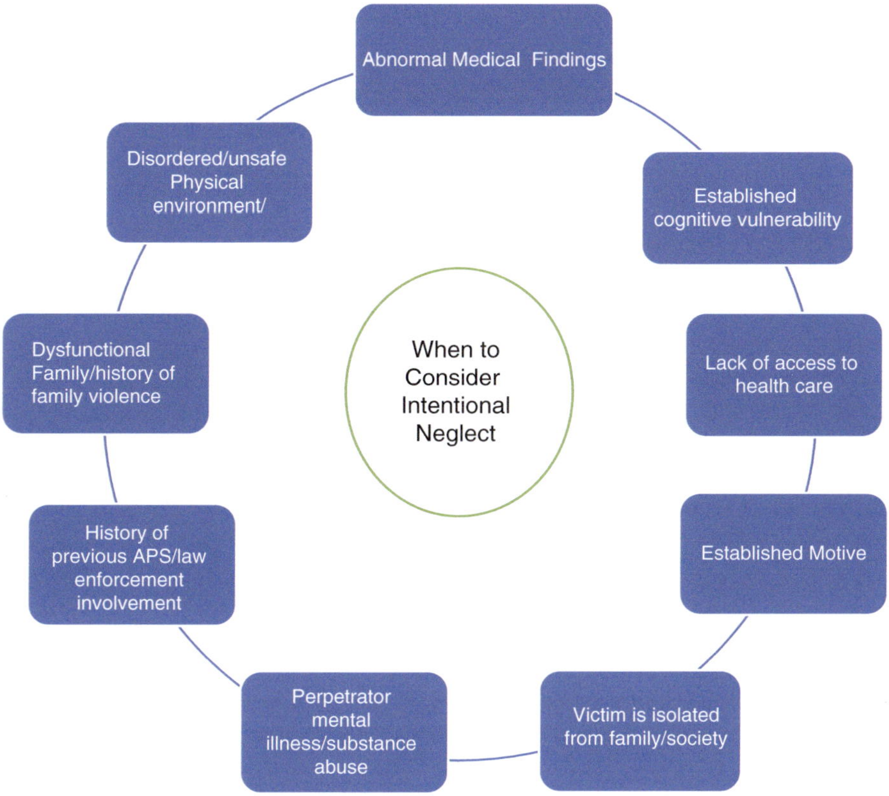

Fig. 7.1 When to consider criminal neglect

Case Discussion

After reviewing all the historical data and considering the rubric postulated in the diagram the practitioner can make a more informed decision about whether the case requires reporting to APS or to law enforcement for further evaluation of criminality. Although any one factor illustrated above may not constitute criminality, when more than one factor is present, concern for intentional neglect should increase. Working with social workers is crucial for the healthcare professional as they are skilled in evaluating and reporting cases to authorities. Depending on your state's laws, however, the fact that a case suggests criminality does not necessarily determine whether it must be reported or prosecuted. Most states require reporting even in less severe cases of neglect.

Abnormal Physical Findings

Ms S. had many of the hallmarks of neglect as described above, most notably dehydration, malnutrition, and extensive, poorly cared for, and infected pressure ulcers.

Cognitive Vulnerability

Ms S. had documented progressive cognitive impairment and clearly had significant physical vulnerability as well. She was bedbound for several months prior to death making her completely dependent on her son, for care for Activities of Daily Living (ADL's), nutrition, and comfort. No formal capacity evaluation was ever carried out as she'd had no recent contact with the medical system. Her son described her as significantly impaired and unable to care for herself. Hospital Emergency Department (ED) recorded significant cognitive impairment after a fall.

Access to Medical Care s

Ms S. last saw her primary care physician 2.5 years prior to her death, at which point follow-up was strongly recommended in 6 weeks. Her son was present at that visit but he did not comply with the PCP's recommendations. Prior to this, Ms S had been interested in her medical care and had accepted recommended surgeries and treatments. Since Ms S. did not come for follow-up appointments, her physician could not continue prescribing medications and she therefore had no medications for the past 2 years.

Six months prior to her death, Ms. S. had a fall out of bed and was evaluated in an ED by Orthopedics with recommendations to follow up in 4 weeks. She did not appear for her follow-up visit. Attempts made to send services into the home and offers for long-term care placements were declined by the patient's son. The medical findings clearly document three hallmarks of neglect: dehydration, malnutrition, and pressure ulcers. She had multiple pressure ulcers in advanced stages that had been poorly cared for, resulting in osteomyelitis of her sacral region.

Unsafe Environment

Ms S. had spent most of her time in bed over the last 6 months. Her room was cluttered and cold; her nutrition consisted of bananas and orange juice and an occasional candy bar; she was incontinent of bowel and bladder and found in soiled clothing. She did not have a proper mattress to protect her skin from breakdown and there were several bags of soiled bedclothes in her bedroom when EMS arrived. There were bottles of antiseptic and bug spray in her room. Her son reported cleaning her pressure ulcers with hydrogen peroxide and rubbing alcohol.

Motive

Although Ms S. had a long history of regularly seeking medical care, when questioned by police, her son claimed his mother did not want to go to the doctor and he was following her wishes. At the same time, the son admitted his mother would have hallucinations and think that his father—who had died years earlier—was in the room with her. Her son further admitted in questioning that he believed she suffered from dementia. As the facts of the case came to light, it became clear that the son preferred to continue living off his mother's income than to find meaningful employment. Her son chose to continue living his comfortable lifestyle rather than divert his mother's income to a care facility or in-home care for her.

Victim-Perpetrator Relationship

Ms S.'s son was an engineer. Over the years, their relationship had been amicable. He had sporadic jobs over the years but had not worked since Ms S. moved to Washington to live with him 3 years before her death. The household was supported by Ms S.'s Social Security income and small pension. Her son had no significant income. He had casual friends he saw frequently at the local bar but spent most of his time at home in his bedroom in the basement of the house where he would gamble on-line. In the last few months of Ms S.'s life, her son would hear her calling out, to which he responded by putting in earplugs. Their neighbors also heard Ms S.; they contacted their landlord, who contacted her son who said things were taken care of. Then they closed their windows.

Social Isolation

Ms S. was entirely dependent on her son for her nutrition, hydration, medical care, and all other personal needs. She was isolated and had no access to a phone. The television in her room didn't work. On the very rare occasion when she had visitors, they were almost always friends of her son's.

Considerations for Prosecutors

Because the system of aging services in this country is inadequate, criminal neglect of older adults is difficult to prosecute. When the system as a whole fails an older adult, then prosecuting the individual caregiver is often impossible, and almost always inappropriate. Those cases that are prosecutable tend to be ones where the system did respond properly—at least somewhat—and the caregiver, as in her sons and Ms S.'s case, was capable of providing proper care or of making proper decisions for the older adult but chose to profit financially rather than obtain the needed care for the dependent person. Had Ms S's PCP detected and reported suspicions of abuse the outcome of this case might have been very different.

In the case of Ms S., her son was charged with Manslaughter in the First Degree, recklessly causing the death of another person. His case went to trial, and he was found guilty of Manslaughter in the Second Degree, causing the death of another person with criminal negligence. He served a sentence of 39 months in prison.

Prosecutors need medical records to have the information they need to make proper and ethical decisions to charge criminal neglect. Typically, in a neglect case, an experienced prosecutor will obtain all relevant records from all health care providers seen by the victim in the last 5 years or more. They will also obtain pharmacy records. Only by closely examining a patient's complete medical history can prosecutors fully understand whether criminal neglect has occurred.

Because these cases are inherently medical in nature, the participation of health care providers is crucial. Experienced elder abuse prosecutors need to consult with health care providers in making their charging decisions in neglect cases, and employ health care providers as expert witnesses in cases on which they file charges. In addition, the primary care provider, physicians, and nurses who treated the victim during, the prior to and after the neglect, as well as hospital social workers, may also become witnesses at trial. Physicians and other healthcare professionals who treated the victim or who are hired as experts may be asked to testify on subjects such as the cause of the victim's symptoms and injuries, the degree of pain they would have suffered, what care should have been provided them, and their degree of cognitive impairment. Without their cooperation, prosecutors would be left to make decisions on these cases on their own, inevitably resulting in uninformed and potentially unethical charging decisions. Health care professionals are encouraged to assist prosecutors with these cases so that proper decisions can be made.

Prosecutors must take care, when presented with a case in which neglect charges may be filed, that such charges should be filed. Sometimes, social and economic issues will arise that make it clear that, even though neglect occurred, the victim, who had capacity, refused to go to the hospital due to legitimate concerns about the impact of his or her hospitalization on her family caregivers. In other situations, it may be clear that the victim had cognitive capacity and freely chose to die at home rather than go to the hospital or a long-term care facility. To assess the various ethical issues that can arise in cases of possible criminal neglect, determining the victim's cognitive capacity, any impediments they may have experienced to obtaining care, their history of seeking and accepting medical care and any possible financial motives of the caregiver, are essential. In making these decisions, too, the assistance of experienced and knowledgeable health care providers is of vital importance.

Key Points

1. Neglect assumes that the victim is mentally or physically unable to perform the basic daily tasks to maintain their physical and mental health and is reliant on the caregiver to provide those services. Determining victims cognitive status and clarifying who has assumed the role of caregiver is crucial to moving forward with a case.
2. Physical and laboratory findings in neglect cases can frequently overlap with normal changes of aging making criminal prosecution challenging.
3. Criminal neglect is a serious charge that requires integrating information from multiple sources to create a full mosaic of the victim's experience and to ensure that all aspects of the situation are being considered. Completing that mosaic requires cooperation of the health care provider, social service agencies, APS and the criminal justice system.
4. Assessing intent to do harm cannot be directly known — it is inferred by careful review of past and recent behaviors of the caregiver, i.e., how they manage the victims health issues, compliance with victims expressed wishes, financial motives etc.
5. Pressure ulcers, although often seen in neglect cases, can occur even with excellent care and should not be immediately assumed to reflect neglect-criminal or otherwise.
6. Respecting victims wishes to remain home and avoid medical care is their right while they retain capacity. When and if capacity is lost and pain and suffering ensue, the caregiver's responsibility is to make decisions that allow the individual to have adequate pain control and to die with dignity.

References

1. Lachs MS, Pillemer K. Elder abuse. Lancet. 2004;364(9441):1263–72.
2. Berman J, Lachs MS. Under the Radar: New York State Elder Abuse Prevalence Study: self-reported prevalence and documented case surveys. Report prepared by Lifespan of Greater Rochester, Inc., Weill Cornell Medical Center of Cornell University, New York City Department for the Aging; 2011.
3. Yon Y, Mikton C. The prevalence of self-reported elder abuse among in community settings: a systematic review and meta-analysis. Trauma Violence Abuse. 2019;20(2):245–59.
4. Heisler CJ. Elder abuse and the criminal justice system: new awareness, new responses. Generations J San Francisco. 2000;24:52–8.
5. Connecticut State Law (CGS17a-412 and 17b-450) Elder neglect.

6. Bond M, Butler K. Elder abuse and neglect. Clin Geriatr Med. 2013;29(1):257–73. Copyright © 2013.
7. Mazzotti MC, Fais P, et al. When the hidden issue of elder abuse leads to death: do not neglect elder neglect. Am J Forensic Med Pathol. 2022;43:60–5.
8. Collins K. Elder maltreatment: a review. Arch Pathol Lab Med. 2006;130(9):1290–6. https://doi.org/10.5858/2006-130-1290-EMAR.
9. Acierno R, Hernandez MA, Amstadter AB, et al. Prevalence and correlates of emotional, physical, sexual, and financial abuse and potential neglect in the United States: the National Elder Mistreatment Study. Am J Public Health. 2010:292–7.
10. (RCW 9A. 08.010(1)(c).) Washington state law reference.
11. Gross C, et al. Clinical indicators of dehydration severity in elderly patients. J Emerg Med. 1992;10:267–74.
12. Collins KA, Howe J. Elder abuse. In: Forensic and legal medicine. Boca Raton: CRC Press; 2023. p. 411–20.
13. Ayus AJ, et al. Abnormalities of water metabolism in the elderly. Semin Nephrol. 1996;16:277–88.
14. Mandal AK, Saklayen MG, Hillman NM, et al. Predictive factors for high mortality in hypernatremic patients. Am J Emerg Med. 1997;15:130–2.
15. Mandal AK, Saklayen MG, et al. Predictive factors for high mortality in hypernatremic patients. Am J Emerg Med. 1997;15:130–2.
16. Warren L, et al. The burden and outcomes associated with dehydration in the elderly, 1191. Am J Public Health. 1994;84:1265–9.
17. Collins KA, Presnell SE. Elder neglect and the pathophysiology of aging. Am J Forensic Med Pathol. 2007;28(2):157–62.
18. Lachs MS, Otto J. Elder abuse roundtable: detection and diagnosis; what are the forensic markers for identifying physical and psychological signs of elder abuse and neglect? National Institute of Justice; 2000.
19. Dyer CB, Connelly MT, et al. The clinical and medical forensics of elder abuse and neglect. In: Bonnie RJ Research Council (US) Panel to Review Risk and Prevalence of Elder Abuse and Elder Neglect. Elder mistreatment: abuse, neglect and exploitation in aging America. National Academies Press. 2003.
20. Ottaviani S, Rondanina E, et al. Multi-dimensional-based prediction of pressure ulcers development and severity in hospitalized frail oldest old: a retrospective study. Clin Interv Aging. 2024;19:1509–17.

Suggested Reading

LoFaso V, Rosen T. Medical and laboratory indicators of elder abuse and neglect. Clin Geriatr. 2014;30(4):713–28.

Lachs MS, Williams CS, O'Brien S, et al. The mortality of elder mistreatment. JAMA. 1998;280:428–32.

Kim L, Mitchell S, Dyer C. Do medical examiners determine elder mistreatment as a cause of death? Forensic Sci Med Pathol. 2007;3:9–13.

Chapter 8
Self-Neglect

Robert Abrams and Richard Machemer

Part 1: Self-Neglect

Introduction

The term "self-neglect" encompasses a range of potentially harmful behaviors, of which refusal of needed services is at the core.

Self-neglect is an imprecisely defined clinical entity but one that can be meaningful, even determinative, in the lives of older people.

The case below was brought to the attention of a geriatrics medical home-visit program by a community social service agency. The agency had been contacted by the client's landlord for concerns about the state of her apartment and the safety of other residents.

Case Presentation

Ms. A was a 78-year-old single woman who lived with her cat in a one-bedroom apartment. She lived there alone for 45 years. In the past Ms. A. had achieved some success in the art world as a sculptor. Her forte was the creation of miniature

R. Abrams (Retired)(✉)
Department of Psychiatry, Weill Cornell Medicine, New York, NY, USA
e-mail: rabrams@med.cornell.edu

R. Machemer (Retired)
St. John Fisher University, Rochester, NY, USA

V. LoFaso, L. Rachmuth (eds.), *Elder Abuse and Neglect*,
https://doi.org/10.1007/978-3-031-97784-8_8

sculptures that depicted objects used in everyday life. A large accumulation of the materials she used for her artwork, including bottle tops, ice-cream sticks, milk cartons and the like, could be seen throughout her apartment. She had collected "everything and anything," leading inevitably to a chaotic, severely congested environment.

In recent years Ms. A. had refused multiple offers by her landlord and social service agencies to help in organizing and cleaning her apartment. Eventually her bedroom became piled floor-to-ceiling with newspapers, boxes, old clothing, pots and pans, and more. The rest of the apartment was equally cluttered, making it difficult and dangerous to enter and exit safely.

Ms. A.'s life was significantly impacted by alcohol addiction. As a young woman, she had been a prolific artist, but as she aged and her alcoholism advanced, she became less productive. When her art no longer sold, Ms. A. continued to drink, but now ever more heavily, often consuming close to a pint of gin every day.

Other health risks also became apparent. Ms. A. had smoked heavily for decades and now suffered from severe emphysema. This condition made walking the short distance from the entrance to the apartment to her couch (the only usably cleared space in her home) labored and exhausting.

When the medical team arrived, they were met by at the door by a thin, frail, poorly groomed older woman. She was markedly short of breath on minimal exertion. Alcohol was noted on her breath. After receiving reassurance that the sole purpose of the visit was for medical care, Ms. A. reluctantly allowed the team to enter the apartment. A small bench was cleared for one member of the team to sit while the others remained standing. The client herself sat on her couch, which was laden with cat hair and dust and had multiple cigarettes burn marks. The cat appeared to be in good health and well fed.

During the visit by the medical care team, a Psycho-Social History was conducted:

Ms. A. was born in New York where she has lived her entire life. She has one sister in California from whom she is estranged. She never married although she spoke wistfully of several relationships she had as a younger woman. She has no children. She described an emotionally traumatic childhood with repeated reference to an "overly strict" mother and verbally abusive father with an explosive and unpredictable temper. Both parents were alcoholic.

The client smoked since she was 20. She drank moderately and socially until she reached her 60s, at which time she began using alcohol increasingly to assuage feelings of loneliness.

She had Medicare.

As noted above, her landlord had tried to work with her to allow her to stay in her apartment, contacting community social service agencies offering to help with cleaning her apartment and managing the disorder. She declined any interventions suggested. More recently her smoke alarm went off after she fell asleep with a lit cigarette, causing a small fire on her couch. Deeply concerned about this incident and the risks it entailed to both the client and her neighbors, the landlord concluded that he must now consider eviction.

Findings of the Geriatric Home-Visit Team:

The apartment had a marked odor of urine. Empty gin bottles were piled high in the kitchen sink. Clutter was everywhere, as described above.

General: The client was a thin, frail, pale woman. She had a productive cough and was notably short of breath as she moved about the apartment. She was dressed in stained sweatpants and a tee shirt, both too large for her small frame. There was a smell of alcohol on her breath.

Vitals: BP 110/70 P-98. O2 Sat 93%.

PERRLA-conjunctival pallor

HEENT: Dentition was poor with several missing teeth. Thyroid nodule. No bruits

Lungs-Coarse, decreased breath sounds throughout. Occasional wheeze. No crackles

Heart- RRR;2/6 systolic murmur at apex

Abdomen- soft non-tender, non-distended

Extremities: no edema. Long thick mycotic toenails

Neurological-Cranial nerves were intact 2–12. Alert and oriented × 3.

Some short-term memory deficits on recall testing. Repetitive. She appeared anxious but not distinctly sad or tearful, and she denied suicidal feelings or intention. Insight was lacking but she was not delusional or otherwise psychotic. After much hesitation she acknowledged that the apartment was in "sorry condition," but was unable or unwilling to appreciate the safety implications, either for herself or others.

Self-Neglect Overview

"Refusal" may well be the operational word in self-neglect. The services declined or avoided may include medical care, as well as help with financial management, meal preparation, personal hygiene and maintenance of a clean and healthful environment. While not all self-neglecters refuse services, and some accept help partially or reluctantly, the more severe manifestations of self-neglect tend to be associated with a person's history of intervention refusal.

In a broader definition, self-neglect is the "inability or refusal to meet one's own basic needs as accepted by societal norms and is characterized by losses in physical, psychological and social domains" [1].

The aspect of "inability" can thus be added to that of "refusal." However, if the inability to maintain oneself in a healthy manner is the result of advanced cognitive impairment, the neglect may cease to become "self-neglect" and may be more accurately characterized as a failure of oversight for an impaired individual, or as abuse, abandonment, neglect or exploitation by others [2]. At the other end of the cognitive ability spectrum, the definition of self-neglect proposed by the National Centers of Elder Abuse also excludes some conscious, voluntary decisions by mentally competent adults [3].

Consequences of Self-Neglect in Old Age

Whatever the fine points of its definition as a clinical entity, self-neglect can be especially consequential for older individuals. Even if it is under-reported and its prevalence not well established, self-neglect by older persons has become a problem of public health dimensions [4]. It is associated with multiple adverse health outcomes, frequent hospitalizations [5, 6]; malnutrition [2]; enhanced mortality risk [7]; depression and exacerbation of other pre-existing mental health conditions [8, 9]; and misuse of prescription medications [10].

The collateral effects of self-neglect are naturally greater in old age. It has been proposed that older persons with self-neglect comprise a distinctly vulnerable group given the range and severity of their risks for poor health outcomes [1, 11]. There is abundant data to support this proposition. To cite just a few such findings: Emergency department use among older self-neglecters has been found to be substantially greater than among non-self-neglecters of similar age, the difference increasing proportionally with severity of self-neglect; and a statistically significant parallel relationship between the degree of geriatric self-neglect and rates of hospital readmission has also been reported [6].

In addition to these specific relationships between self-neglect and hospital usage, the longer-term effects of self-neglect impact health and well-being in old age more generally and in a wide social network. Neglect of the home and one's immediate environment, particularly when exacerbated by hoarding, can lead to the potential for fires and harm to individuals other than the hoarder himself. In addition, use of community based medical and social services are increased, as described in Ms. A.'s case.

Moreover, the frustration and despair experienced by neighbors, family members and friends of self-neglecters should be considered a significant social outcome of this behavior. In the U.S., self-neglect has been found to be the most frequent report received by state agencies on aging mandated to investigate abuse, neglect and exploitation of adults. This trend was further exacerbated by the Covid pandemic [12].

Self-Neglect as a Geriatric Syndrome: Predictors and Risk Factors

Geriatric self-neglect is frequently seen in the context of pre-existing physical and cognitive frailty. Self-neglect is also found in situations where the affected person lives alone, is estranged or geographically distant from family members, or is for other reasons isolated. These age-related medical and social conditions together represent a starting point of vulnerability, contributing to the subsequent downstream health risks of self-neglect for older people. Nearly all of the key predisposing factors for self-neglect, including alcohol dependence, are illustrated in the case of Ms A.

Geriatric Mental Status Predictors of Self-Neglect

In an early study of the epidemiology of self-neglect in an older adult population, Abrams et al. [8] extracted data from a cohort of community residents in New Haven who were 65 years of age and older. The authors found that persons with clinically significant depressive symptoms and cognitive impairment were more likely than others to experience self-neglect. Separately and together, depression and cognitive impairment were critical components of a combined model for predicting self-neglect.

Consistent with the principal findings from the New Haven investigation, another population-based cohort study, the Chicago Health and Aging Project, also supported age-related changes in mental status as major predictors of self-neglect [4, 6]. These predictors included cognitive decline along a spectrum of severity beginning with loss of executive function and proceeding through the progressive stages of dementia, as well as a range of symptomatic expressions of anxiety and depression. Late-life depression in its more severe forms, such as the DSM-defined entity of major depressive disorder [13], frequently induces subjective experiences of helplessness and hopelessness that detract from a person's ability to look after self, environment, or both. As will be seen in a subsequent section, other behavioral factors, including certain personality traits or symptoms, may contribute specifically to the etiology of hoarding.

Demographic Factors

In addition to mental health factors, the larger predictive model from the New Haven study included male gender, older age, annual income less than $15,000, living alone, history of hip fracture, and history of stroke [8]. Older age, race, gender, and socioeconomic status represented by level of education, were also emphasized in the Chicago Health and Aging Project. Among other Chicago Project findings, Black older adults (men, 13.2%; and women, 10.9%) had higher prevalences of self-neglect than white older adults (men, 2.4%; and women, 2.6%); and all adults with less than high school educations had a higher prevalence of self-neglect than their peers with more extensive educations [4].

Physical disability, particularly hip fracture, was observed in both the New Haven and Chicago cohort studies [4, 6, 8] to be another age-related predictor of self-neglect. Decline in the ability to independently perform daily tasks, especially when associated with cerebrovascular accidents, was also considered under the category of physical disability in these data.

It should be noted that some of the clinical, as opposed to demographic, risk factors associated with self-neglect in older individuals are difficult to distinguish from *consequences* of the self-neglecting behaviors. Nutritional deficiencies, for example, or untreated medical or psychiatric conditions including substance abuse could be appreciated equally well as cause or effect.

The Effect of Traumatic Experiences in Life

For a deeper understanding of the behavioral underpinnings of self-neglecting behaviors in older adults, Lien et al. [9] elicited unstructured narratives in a sample of cognitively intact self-neglecting volunteers. Content analysis of the narratives revealed patterns of traumatic experience, including loss, separation and abandonment; severe lifelong mental illness; repeated refusal of medical interventions; and history of substance abuse.

In the Lien study, the prominence of traumatic experiences earlier in life with a self-neglecting dénouement in old age represented a novel finding that may be of considerable importance if replicated and might also suggest new approaches to intervention.

The stressful or traumatic life events reported by older people are likely to be impactful, even if they differ from those experienced by younger adults. In addition, events in later life typically include the death of a spouse or partner, or any other change in circumstances that results in a person living alone and can also have a significant impact. Living alone itself deprives a vulnerable older person of the help of a spouse or adult child, and can produce a "bell jar" phenomenon in which there is no check on one's perceptions or reasoning, in some instances allowing personal eccentricities to lapse into self-neglecting behaviors.

After considering all of the predictive factors for self-neglect mentioned here, one is left with the impression that old age itself may be the most important, because many of the individual factors have been determined to be independently age-related [14].

Recognizing the close relationship of self-neglect, including both its risks and outcomes, to aging, Pavlou and Lachs [5] concluded that self-neglect is a largely geriatric syndrome. More recently, but in the same direction, Pickens et al. [1, 15] created a comprehensive conceptual model for self-neglect in which the more severe forms are recognized as a condition that predominantly affects an older population.

Assessment of Geriatric Self-Neglect in Research and Practice

Estimates of the reach and clinical impact of self-neglect in the geriatric population have been impeded by the absence of a universally accepted diagnostic standard for the condition. Notably, the latest guideline of mental health diagnoses, the DSM-5-Text Revision published in 2022 [13], includes a detailed entry for Hoarding Disorder but no mention of the broader, more clinically diverse condition of self-neglect.

Important questions about the diagnosis of self-neglect therefore remain unresolved. First, are there any exclusions to making the diagnosis? As mentioned previously, severe cognitive impairment might contribute one such exclusion. Then, in such cases of advanced dementia, the question referenced earlier arises again: Should behaviors related to cognitive loss be deemed self-neglect, or should self-neglect be limited to individuals with at most mild-to-moderate dementia, i.e., those whose self-neglecting behaviors can be linked to an intentional, if unwise, choice?

In a thoughtful review, Dong [14], considering the diagnostic boundaries of self-neglect, suggested that assessment of decision-making capacity might be more relevant than cognitive screening alone to case identification of self-neglect. If self-neglect is to be considered a conscious individual choice, a certain level of decisional ability might then be required to make the diagnosis.

Nevertheless, prevalence estimates of geriatric self-neglect are likely to be affected by the level of cognitive impairment allowed for inclusion, with studies of individuals who are more than moderately cognitively impaired likely to yield higher prevalences [15]. If a DSM diagnosis for self-neglect could be developed based on expert consensus, agreement on the question of how large a net of inclusion should be applied would at least provide a uniformly accepted starting point.

Scales and Inventories Used in Self-Neglect Research

The absence of a set of standardized criteria for the categorical diagnosis of self-neglect has given rise to the creation of several scales to establish the presence and measure the extent of such behaviors [16]. Despite some content overlap, these scales have been predicated on differing assumptions, and they tend to weigh the same behaviors differently according to importance [2]. Since no single scale is suitable for all purposes, protocols may be selected for research studies according to what is emphasized in a particular inquiry.

Several of the presently available research instruments rely on a dimensional design, associating the phenomenon of self-neglect with scores at a particular threshold [1, 16, 17]. In that way they can be used both to establish the presence or absence of self-neglect generally, and also estimate the extent or severity of such behaviors. However, comparing studies using different measurement schemes is inevitably confusing, even if the same domains are being assessed. What one team of researchers deems to rise to the level of categorical self-neglect may not comport with that of their colleagues working elsewhere.

Also, the problem of validation of these assessment tools might never be satisfactorily resolved in the absence of a universally accepted "gold standard" for self-neglect. Lacking such consensus, researchers are compelled to find their own gold standards; when creating the Abrams Geriatric Self-Neglect Scale (AGSS) [2], for example, the investigators relied on an independent expert panel of physicians with American Board of Psychiatry and Neurology Certification in Geriatric Psychiatry to create a list of criteria they agreed to be essential to the concept of self-neglect in old age.

A different, but equally daunting impediment to diagnosis of self-neglect in both research and clinical practice is the propensity of self-neglecters to minimize or deny their self-neglecting behaviors, so that their own accounts may have limited value. It may therefore be necessary to interview family members or friends for purposes of corroboration. Psychiatric expertise may be also be required in the assessment process, given the mental health etiologies of much self-neglecting behavior. Although not a mandatory component of most self-neglect assessment scales, many evaluations would be incomplete without on-site home inspections to supplement reports from other sources.

It is beyond the scope of this chapter to summarize, let alone compare the psychometric properties of all extant self-neglect scales, but it would be of interest to briefly describe the design and domains of those frequently cited in the self-neglect literature. The following is intended only as a representative sample:

The Self-Neglect Severity Scale (SSS)

The SSS [17] organizes questions by category: personal hygiene; cognitive, health and safety issues; and environmental assessment. The related SN-37 contains 37 items organized into 5 more abstract behavioral factors seen as contributors to self-neglect: environment, social networks, emotional and behavioral lability, health avoidance and self-determinism.

The Kohlman Evaluation of Living (KELS)

The KELS [18] emphasizes basic and instrumental activities of daily living, and has been used effectively in guardianship hearings to establish ability of a person to live independently.

The Abrams Geriatric Self-Neglect Scale (AGSS)

The AGSS [2] is designed to assess self-neglect specifically in older populations along six domains: management of prescription medications, intended as a proxy for adherence to *all* medical attention; personal care; nutrition; environment/housing, under which the feature of hoarding is subsumed if present; financial stewardship; and socialization.

In general, the AGSS and others are thought to represent conceptual expansions of the SSS, the instrument that may be closest to a "gold standard" in this field.

Hoarding Disorder

> "If there is nothing you can share with other people, try to be close to Things; they will not abandon you". From (Rainer Maria) Rilke's Letter to a Young Poet: The Sixth Letter

Since the behavior of hoarding can be so dramatic in presentation, especially in severe cases, it can be viewed as the "public face" of self-neglect in both geriatric and general adult populations. Hoarding is in fact the subject of much public discussion across all media. Since 2013 it has been the only sub-category of self-neglect that has been included in the American Psychiatric Association's Diagnostic and Statistical Manual (DSM) series [19]. Like established mental disorders, but *unlike* most domains of self-neglect, Hoarding Disorder is a discrete single entity that is readily and unmistakably identifiable. Hoarding activity has been described in detail and even staged using various schemes [20], with the severity of symptoms reflecting both the *quantity* of hoarded objects and the social and psychological *effects* of the behavior. For all of these reasons, hoarding is the only presentation of self-neglect that has been given a separate section in this chapter.

The definition in DSM-5-Text Revision of Hoarding Disorder is characterized by "persistent difficulty in discarding or parting with possessions, regardless of their actual value, as a result of a strong perceived need to save the items and distress associated with discarding them." The hoarded items are typically not needed and often remain with their packaging unopened; they produce clutter that can restrict the use of critical areas of the home, for example, making kitchens, bathrooms and sleeping areas unusable. Many individuals with this disorder are intensely focused on the acquisition and collection of these unneeded, unused objects.

As with most DSM entities, to make a definitive diagnosis, several general conditions that characterize mental disorders must be met. These requirements stipulate that the hoarding behavior must cause either significant distress to the individual or impairment in social or occupational functioning; the behavior cannot be attributable to another cause or condition; and it cannot be better explained by the symptoms of another mental disorder.

In the DSM conception of hoarding, other mental disorders, including psychotic, mood, personality and neurocognitive conditions, must be ruled out as causative. However, these other entities may still exist comorbidly with hoarding disorder. Comorbidity also applies to various personality disorder traits, not necessarily disorders, that have been associated with hoarding and may predispose individuals to it; these traits include obsessionality, avoidance, procrastination or disorganization not directly related to dementia.

The relationship between hoarding and obsessional personality traits may be particularly important. In fact, the DSM diagnosis of hoarding is classified alongside Obsessive Compulsive Disorder, and the two entities have been shown to involve similar cognitive difficulties, such as executive dysfunction, delays in set shifting, spatial planning, and overall cognitive flexibility. At the same time, however, the clinical presentations of Hoarding Disorder and Obsessive Compulsive Disorder are distinctly different [21].

DSM also includes "specifiers" that describe the presence or absence of personal insight into the hoarding behavior, and the presence or absence of excessive acquisition of objects, the latter being a feature of the majority of cases. In persons with excessive acquisition, it is noted that some hoard animals as well as inanimate objects.

Is Hoarding Disorder actually a geriatric condition, in the way that the other manifestations of self-neglect have been presented in this chapter? The condition is chronic, generally emerging in young adulthood when adolescents begin to live on their own, and typically worsening by late middle and advanced age [22]. Prevalence estimates tend to show a predominance in the over-65 age range. The prevalences for men and women are thought to be roughly comparable.

It is also important to note that in clinical experience, hoarding disorder does not generally exist alone, but is found in concert with other signs of self-neglect. Hoarding is not precisely synonymous with broader definitions of self-neglect, but the behavior of hoarding, if advanced, precludes attention to one's physical and emotional health and leads to increased social isolation.

The chronicity and symptomatic worsening over time of hoarding behaviors appear to contribute to the muted response to intervention and the largely negative prognostic outlook [22]. For clinicians and social service agencies, interventions therefore require patience, tolerance, and ability to persist despite considerable frustration and recidivism. In the end, the threat of legal sanctions such as involuntary major cleaning, dispossession and eviction hangs over many cases.

Several associated features have been highlighted in recent studies of hoarding, including inconsistent regulation of emotion, intolerance of uncertainty and distress, and difficulties around the experience of attachment [23]. These discoveries have led to the development of novel psychotherapeutic treatments for hoarding, including group-based therapy and approaches that use a cognitive-behavioral model [24–26]. These interventions appear to be heavily dependent on individual motivation and tend to be more effective in milder cases. Simply addressing social isolation with the intention of gradually replacing objects with people, appears to be helpful for some, but not all, hoarders.

However, as indicated above, the clinical experience in treating Hoarding Disorder with cognitive behavioral approaches and novel interventions has been variably successful. The association of hoarding with executive dysfunction and other early cognitive deficits may contribute to the disappointing intervention outcomes. Also, the putative effects of traumatic events, abandonments, and losses in early life on hoarding behavior may be unreachable without in-depth psychological treatments.

Since the ethos of social intervention is to always seek the "least restrictive alternative," dramatic and definitive solutions to self-neglect and hoarding, such as the Heavy Duty Cleaning sometimes involuntarily imposed by Adult Protective Services (APS) organizations in New York State, are relatively infrequent and used only when basic public health conditions are egregiously violated. In a few states agencies like APS, upon whom much of the social burden inevitably falls, may institute emergency involuntary removals and in extreme cases, guardianship [26]. Sometimes these measures are tied to involuntary hospitalization of the individual; however, the circumstances justifying that level of intervention are legally and ethically required to be dire and life-threatening and thus apply only to the most aggravated cases.

Aside from the potential violation of the civil liberties of clients, anecdotal experience reveals that dramatic interventions such as Heavy Duty Cleaning and involuntary removal from one's home can be psychologically injurious and can be regarded as the equivalent of "dynamiting one's external defensive structure" with unknown long-term consequences.

An advantage of the private intervention by "hoarding specialists" is the "luxury of time" that can be used to involve the client directly in the process of discarding unneeded objects. In this writer's own experience, relinquishing objects can entail a prolonged sequence for each object that is close to the trajectory of mourning, so that many such objects cannot be relinquished in a single session; it is a process that has elements of both psychodynamic psychotherapy and grief counseling.

Moreover, if certain vulnerability factors can be identified early in life, a path to meaningful prevention of hoarding might be forged [27]. Such vulnerability might reflect a history of traumatic separations, homelessness, or environmental unpredictability in childhood, affecting lifelong emotional attachments to material possessions.

Clinical Considerations

The initial approach to addressing self-neglect in an older person would be examine for, and manage, any age-related emotional or physical conditions that might explain or shed light on the picture. For example, depression, whether acute or chronic, is inherently syntonic with self-neglect. The despair and hopelessness experienced by individuals with major depression are likely to exacerbate, if not cause, the particular range of behaviors that are relevant here. The same effect can be observed with many medical conditions, especially chronic illnesses that entail fatigue and disability in older persons. A search for related conditions and possible underlying causes of any clinical phenomenon is in fact a core axiom of geriatric medicine.

What follows those initial examinations and treatments is less straightforward. Tenacious refusal of services or interventions appears to be the norm rather than the exception among self-neglecters; self-neglecters are not, by definition, voluntary seekers of help. As suggested earlier, refusal may even be the defining aspect of self-neglect, but if so, aging, with the inevitability of medical conditions, is the principal complicating factor. The fact that the older adult may have avoided health maintenance without consequence is often used by self-neglecters to rationalize the continued refusal of medical interventions. That level of refusal increases health risks as chronic conditions fester untreated [24, 28].

In addition to refusal of services, another barrier to intervention is the lack of motivation for change on the part of older individuals who are self-neglecters. Self-neglecters are often impervious to the adverse conditions and environments they have created for themselves, and even if they are aware, they tend to develop a high tolerance for disorder, clutter, odors, or filth. Some have lived alone for many years, and as noted earlier, living alone and social isolation are factors that serve to increase and perpetuate self-neglect because no sustained challenges are posed to the individual's *modus operandi.*

Perhaps the most difficult situations confronted by social service agencies arise when the older adult involved appears to have decisional capacity but is living in conditions that profoundly threaten their safety as well as that of others. In such situations, considerations of safety prevail, but there are gradations of safety that must be considered [29, 30]. Since refusal of services is so often at the heart of geriatric self-neglect, standardized assessment of decision-specific capacity is an important tool that can be used by organizations such as APS before resorting to the final arbiter of judicial rulings [31].

Self-neglecters are not necessarily expected to be insightful about themselves, but if cognitively intact, some will retain the capacity to reason; and so, with time, they might be able to appreciate the consequences of self-neglect that they can see in others and adapt these observations for themselves. This is perhaps the central tenet of many group therapies. Otherwise, those who attend local senior centers may be more willing to accept the opinions and standards of peers than of authority figures. However, peer-group discussions, whether in group therapy settings or informal gatherings, have not been studied extensively, either for hoarding or for self-neglecting behaviors generally.

The sparse existing research on intervention for older self-neglecters emphasizes the need for patience and for social worker-client relationships that highlight the client's development of trust as the mutative element. Whether or not healthcare systems should support individualized interventions that incur large expenditures of time, effort and financial resources remains an open question.

A substantial contributor to the social cost of self-neglect in older adults is the onus of responsibility placed on the individual's family members or concerned friends. This burden includes the difficulty of confronting the client's resistance to their efforts to help and when necessary taking on the responsibility of establishing a legally recognized protective status. But even in instances of established guardianship, there are limits to what the self-neglecting older adults can be compelled to do involuntarily.

All considered, there is nothing efficient or cost-effective about creating ethical interventions for geriatric self-neglect. Each client is a case series of one, requiring a treatment plan designed specifically for himself and taking into account a set of circumstances unique to the individual.

Key Points

1. Self-neglect is a broad, inclusive entity that largely, although not exclusively, affects older people. It involves multiple symptom areas, including failure to seek adequate medical care, maintain personal hygiene and a healthful environment, sustain proper nutrition, and manage financial resources.
2. Refusal of needed services may be the defining feature of geriatric self-neglect and is usually the impetus for medical or legal intervention.
3. Hoarding Disorder is a specific subcategory of self-neglect, the only one that is recognized by the American Psychiatric Association's latest Diagnostic and Statistical Manual. Other areas of self-neglect are assessed by the various scales designed for use in research studies and clinical settings.

4. At advanced levels of cognitive impairment, self-neglect becomes involuntary and therefore is likely to represent neglect or exploitation by others. A practical way of determining the boundaries of self-neglect in a given situation is to assess a client's decision-specific capacity to refuse a service that is deemed necessary for that person's well-being.
5. Intervention begins with considering all possible psychiatric and medical causes for the self-neglecting behavior and addressing them to the extent possible. Following that, the diagnosis of self-neglect and/or Hoarding Disorder should be reviewed, if necessary augmenting patient self-report with corroborative informants and home assessments.

   Then, cognitive-behavioral treatment paradigms can be applied, but their effectiveness has not been well established. Efforts to minimize social isolation and to encourage peer interaction have shown some promise. Individual coaching for hoarding behavior can be effective but is expensive and time-consuming. All such interventions need to be tailored to the personal requirements of individual cases. In the end, legal sanctions mandating involuntary removal from one's environment or guardianship are solutions of last resort used to assure safety when all else has failed.

Part 2: Self-Neglect

Introduction

This section will describe the principles of normal biological aging, the need to distinguish between biological processes in aging and the manifestations of aging, the functional approach to aging (successful, usual, and pathological), and changes in homeostasis that occur during the aging process. The question remains whether self-neglect is a biologically caused phenomenon or is the result of an adverse environment that has compromised and distorted the biological function of an individual. It appears that the latter—an adverse environment that affects the manifestations of the biological process of aging—is the more likely situation.

Self-Neglect Biological Overview

The case study in Part 1 presents a complicated but all-too-common look at the impact on self-neglect on the life of a person who is older. Ms. A is exhibiting a variety of behaviors that are putting her at great personal risk and potentially putting her neighbors at great risk. This geriatric syndrome—it's predictors, risk factors, general considerations, and approach to the case present a wide array of issues that need to be addressed. One of the factors often cited as a risk factor for self-neglect is "old age." What is there about being older that increases the chances of self-neglect manifesting in an individual? Is it "old age" per se that causes self-neglect? Or is it the numerous changes, diseases, dysfunctions that may occur with older age but that are not caused by the aging process, that put the person at risk for experiencing self-neglect? There is an additional question one can raise—what brought about this functional state? Not every person who is older exhibits self-neglect characteristics much less to the degree seen with Ms. A. The long-debated nature vs. nurture discussion and controversy again comes to the fore. It seems unlikely that the biological process of aging directly causes self-neglect (unless the biological drive to self-neglect occurs so late that the individual dies due to some other cause, before self-neglect can manifest.) Were self-neglect biologically caused, everyone who lives long enough would develop this geriatric syndrome. Those who did not exhibit this syndrome would not have done so because they died before the self-neglect could manifest. However, are there biological changes that could put the individual at greater risk of developing self-neglect? Would these biological factors be more likely to manifest if they occurred within an environment that's associated with a greater risk of developing this syndrome? We know that the environment in which an individual lives and functions has a dramatic impact on the manifestations of aging. The social determinants of health (SDOH) and commercial determinants of health (CDOH) affect how the aging process "appears" to be taking place. Do they influence aging by altering genetic activity? Do they have impact in persons who are biologically-vulnerable"—those persons who have a lower reserve capacity or lessened degrees of resilience? Long-term high-level stress, and the attendant significantly elevated levels of cortical steroids is known to reduce cell numbers in certain parts of the brain, particularly the hippocampus. Numerous correlations have been drawn between environmental factors in an individual's life and the likelihood of developing self-neglect (as well as the degree of self-neglect). The question remains as to whether there's a specific genotype that in the appropriately negative environment puts the person at risk of developing self-neglect. Or are the biological underpinning, to this disorder simply factors that allow, rather than cause, this syndrome to develop?

This following brief look at the process of aging, the broad functional outcomes of biological aging process, and at the changes that occur in homeostatic regulation with increasing age, may help one to develop a framework from which to better understand the underpinnings of self-neglect.

Self-neglect, as described in Part 1 of this chapter, is "…the inability or refusal to meet one's own basic needs as accepted by societal norms…and is characterized by losses in the physical, psychological, and social domains". The question becomes whether there is some aspect of the basic biological process of aging that contributes to this "inability." For example, one could examine cognitive changes with aging. There is an expected slowing of cognitive function in the latter stages of the life cycle. Is that change sufficient to lead to self-neglect? Or is it only when the cognitive change extends well beyond typical normal changes—as for example in a condition of a dementia or brain injury—that self-neglect becomes a possibility? Or might it be that self-neglect brought about by other factors, alters brain function to diminish cognition well beyond normal and this lower cognitive function then exacerbates the self-neglect? It's clear that these environmental influences can alter function and are associated with self-neglect. However, the question remains, is there some age-associated biological change—not disease or dysfunction—in one of the other functional systems in a human—sensory, muscular system, endocrine, immune, e.g.—that brings about this lessened ability or the "inability" to provide self-care? Perhaps it's not a single biological change that's a causative factor for self-neglect. Perhaps it's several biological factors that in combination with each other, initiate a cascade of changes that result in self-neglect. Could the numerous negative attributes of a less-than-appropriate environment in which an individual functions be the trigger to alter the biological process of aging in a way that could then contribute to self-neglect? The poor social determinants of health are known to contribute to the functional changes one sees in self-neglect. But why are some persons resistant to this influence and others not? Is there a difference in how the aging process is taking place in these more resistant (or resilient) individuals? While this is not the focus of this section, one could explore functional changes in each body system to look for changes that are correlated with the behaviors of self-neglect. For example, work is underway to examine changes in neuronal function in specific brain regions that regulate perseverance, exploration and disengagement [32]. Might this approach have impact in humans if such regions can be altered and lead to less perseverance or perhaps more disengagement? These changes could then manifest as behaviors we describe as self-neglect. If these studies (currently done only in mice) can be extended to humans, they may offer us at least a partial explanation for self-neglect. We can't change the genetically driven process of aging at any time in the life cycle. However, we do know that the environment—external and internal psychological in particular—can alter the expression of the genes (through epigenetic changes [33]). One assumes that this is also the situation with genes that may "cause" or be related to causing the aging process. The environment can be changed to lessen the negative impact it has on an individual. It's the gene-environmental interaction that results in what we see in a person during the aging process…the manifestations of aging.

Far too often one assumes that all the changes –expected and disease related— that one finds in persons who are older are biologically-caused changes. It's part of the genetic focus—aging is caused by genes, and nothing can be done to alter it. This then leads us to the three questions about self-neglect and aging. Do the biological changes that occur during aging directly cause self-neglect? Do the biological changes that occur with aging increase the likelihood that self-neglect will occur when an individual lives in a poor environment (from numerous SDOH and CDOH perspectives)? Do the biological changes of aging have essentially nothing to do with causing this syndrome of self-neglect?

To begin this process, one needs to understand that there is a major difference between the biological process of aging (all the changes that happen at the subcellular, cellular, tissue, organ, and organ system level) and the outward manifestations of aging (what is seen in a person who is older). It is not the intent of this section to examine all the aging changes system-by-system and determine how they may impact function. The focus here is on functional aging to see how this may have already impacted Ms. A and will continue to impact her as she continues to age. Finally, we'll look at homeostasis from a functional perspective to help "explain" the wider variability among persons who are older—the heterogeneity of aging. This may help us to better understand the broad process of change in aging that put Ms. A into her current situation of self-neglect. While it would be interesting to explore all the historical factors that may have had an impact on Ms. A's development of self-neglect (a root-cause-analysis), this is not the focus of this section. The focus of this chapter is what can now be done to improve her situation.

What Is Aging

The word aging and the concept of aging often seem very simple—grow chronologically old, experience disease, decline, and eventually die. If one were to ask groups of individuals to describe aging, the response might be something like this: "Aging is growing old, becoming much less functional, developing disease, becoming fully dependent and then dying, all alone, in constant pain, and in an institution." And because it is often assumed that this process is entirely biological, one assumes that there is no control over the outcome of any aspect of aging. Much of this approach originates in the anti-aging "movement" that suggests the aging process is a disease, an "insult", something that "needs" to be "cured" [34, 35]. What is needed is a different mind-set, an altered frame of reference about aging—what it is and how it plays out over a lifetime.

One way to conceptualize what constitutes the aging process is to understand and accept that aging is the series of changes that occur from the moment the egg and sperm come together until the moment the individual dies. Much of what happens in latter stages of the life cycle is a continuation of what began earlier in the life cycle. Late-life changes are a portion of the process of aging, not the entire process. We divide the life cycle into different periods for convenience and because during these time periods—infancy, toddlerhood, youth, teen years, young adult, middle age, older adult—individuals share an array of common characteristics. In this broader and biologically based view of aging, the many of changes that happen through this life course are all considered to be parts of aging. Aging is change, growth, development and striving for maximizing function. Aging is repairing, replacing, renewing cells and tissues. Aging is a functional decline (generally chronologically later in the life cycle). And aging is a process that culminates in death. By accepting the conception-to-death view of aging, one has the perspective that the latter stages and changes develop based on changes that developed in and continue from the previous stages. One is also more likely to avoid the erroneous view that aging is about nothing but decline. In the case of Ms. A, this long-range view would be an additional way to understand what may have brought about her current situation. It is from an understanding of the unfolding of biological aging over this long time period with all its many expressions (growth development, repair, replacement, e.g.) that one may gain better insights into why self-neglect is a major outcome for some persons.

Beyond the narrow view that aging is only late-life changes, one also needs to separate what ones sees in a person who is older—the manifestations, the outward look of aging—from the biological process that drives this process. This distinction requires that one include the impact that the non-biological external environment has on the individual (that also includes the psychological environment and the thought processes occurring in an individual). It's the interaction of the genes of the individual and the environment in which those individual genes functions, that result in what we see—the manifestations. One is not looking directly at the biological changes—those many tens of thousands of changes at the molecular, subcellular, cellular, tissue, organ, and organ system levels. It's the manifestation of aging, the outward appearance of aging, that we see in Ms. A in her current living situation. Has the biological process of aging had an impact on her functional state at this stage in her life? Yes. But which of the changes we see in her function are biological—and probably can't be changed—and which are environmental (that includes disease and dysfunction) and may be changed? There are numerous theories that attempt to account for how the aging process takes place and why the manifestations of aging are what we see. Perhaps the one that is most useful application to the case study and Ms. A is the functional theory of aging, first presented in 1987 by Rowe and Kahn [36, 37].

Functional Model of Aging

The functional theory of Rowe and Kuhn [36, 37] describes a broad perspective from which to view aging and the changes that are a part of the process. This theory focuses on what the individual is able to do and how the interplay of genes and environment affect an individual's function. This functional description of aging divides the outcomes of this interactive process into three categories: successful, usual, and pathological. "Successful" is often viewed as a judgmental term. That is not the intent. Successful used in this functional model is used as a biological term. This approach can be applied at all stages of the life cycle. The focus here is on only the latter stages of that cycle and asks what might have led to Ms. A's current functional state—is it biological changes? Is it environmental changes? Is it environmental impacts on the biological process of aging?

Gene-Environment Interplay Leading to the Manifestations of Aging

Aging is an interaction between the genes (fixed but that show variation in terms of expression due to epigenetic factors) and the environment (changeable) in which the individual functions at all stages in the life cycle. This interplay is what is seen in the person who is older. This is what one assesses when one looks at the function of a person at any age. Rowe and Kahn [36, 37] used terms that one might question today from a bio-gerontological perspective: successful, usual, and pathological with successful being the controversial one. There is a substantial amount of research and resulting literature that's developed around this functional model. This is well beyond the study of this case, but a brief overview is vital to understanding the range of functional states one finds in persons who are chronologically older.

Successful Aging

In this context, successful means positive genes expressed in a positive environment. The outward look of aging, that is, the manifestations of aging, show no signs of clinical disease at least until the mid-to-late 70s. It doesn't mean that there is no clinical disease or never will be any disease. As long as the appearance is not negatively affecting one's overall function, it will have no impact on overall biological function. It's that biological function that remains high and that does not require environmental (or significant medical) compensations. As Rowe and Kahn further elaborated, successful aging is more than an absence of disease. It's more than maintaining high functional abilities, both physical and cognitive. It is those factors and the active engagement with life that result in successful aging. Changes happen; disease can occur. But it's the positive interplay among these three factors—avoiding disease and disability, having high cognitive and physical function, and engaging with life—that describes the way successful aging is manifested in an individual.

Usual Aging

Usual aging could result from neutral genes in a neutral environment; or it could be positive genes in a negative environment. Whatever the combination, there is an obvious decline in function that includes the impact of a disease or diseases or some dysfunction(s). The gene-environmental-disease-dysfunction interactions result in functional changes in that person that are obvious and that can markedly interfere with maintaining a high quality of living experience. These persons continue to function well, continue to experience at least a relatively high quality of living as long as necessary environmental modifications are available and made. One, two, or all three of the realms that define successful aging—avoiding disease and disability, retaining high cognitive and physical function, and engaging with life—are negatively affected in usual aging. Interventions in a vast array of different ways—including medical—are made to lessen the negative impact that the environment (and disease or dysfunction) have on the individual. It's the appropriate environmental compensation (that includes psychological) that must be made and made in whatever way(s) are needed. When this is done, functional abilities can remain high.

Pathological Aging

Persons in the pathological aging realm may have negative genes that are expressed in a negative environment. These individuals require continuing and usually high-level interventions if they are to continue to live. While the "negative genes" cannot be altered, the impact of the larger environment must be addressed and changed to a more positive one if that person is to survive.

Case Discussion

We have no way to determine the "kind" of genes Ms. A has—positive, neutral, or negative. And even if we did, there's no biological way (yet) to change the physical nature of those genes. The expression of the genes can be modified by a variety of the environment factors through the epigenetic process [33, 34]. She may have a gene or genes that put her at greater risk of functional decline if and when "activated" by a particular environment. We don't know which gene or genes, or the degree of environmental triggering is necessary to alter that gene's function. We do know that her environment has been a negative one, a "hostile" one, for a significant portion of her life cycle, perhaps her entire life. That negative environment has directly or indirectly led to the serious changes she's exhibiting at this later stage in her life. We can assess her environment now as was clearly outlined in Part 1. While we don't know specifically what her earlier life was like, one can presume (based on the hoarding as described in Part 1), that changes (may) have occurred very early in her life that were negative. Her actions during her adult years have put her at a significantly higher risk for disease, dysfunction and of dying than would have happened had she been living in a positive or at least a neutral environment. The focus must now be on a variety of environmental interventions that could help enhance Ms. A's present function. Addressing her mental state, and what may be done, about that is the main priority. However, one needs to go well beyond "just" the mental function…as the list of approaches in Part 1 clearly outlines.

Are there specific biological (e.g., genetic) factors that when expressed in a "triggering environment" (one that allows or causes genes to change activity—the epigenetic factors) that could help account for the self-neglect seen later in life? That is, is self-neglect a biologically based or biologically triggered process? Or is self-neglect a result of the early life and continuing environmental challenges that distort the biological compensation and resiliency? These are questions to which we do not yet have satisfactory or complete answers.

There is one final piece of the later-life aging process that's important to understand. It helps one understand why biologically Ms. A's function places her into such a precarious and potential life-death situation. This is biological resilience and the ability to counter the impacts of the environment. The question is what happens to normal function when there is a stress (i.e., any change in function, not simply what is perceived by an individual as "bad") and in what way or ways does this response change as one becomes older? This is the phenomenon of homeostasis—relative functional constancy in a changing environment.

Homeostasis

Homeostasis is a familiar term in the biological world, the environmental world, and the human-made mechanical world. In the biological world, one descriptor of homeostasis is the following: homeostasis, any self-regulating process by which biological systems tend to maintain stability while adjusting to conditions that are optimal for survival. If homeostasis is successful, life continues; if unsuccessful, disaster or death ensues. The stability attained is actually a dynamic equilibrium, in which continuous change occurs yet relatively uniform conditions prevail. The general idea of this self-regulating process was explored by French physiologist Claude Bernard in 1849 and the word *homeostasis* coined by American neurologist and physiologist Walter Bradford Cannon in 1926 [38, 39].

Homeostatic function is seen at all levels in the biological world: the subcellular, the cellular, the tissue, the organ, and the organ system levels. To say that a biological system maintains stability, does not mean that the function doesn't change—it does not mean that the function remains an absolute constant. There is always a pattern of change that is considered normal. When an environmental challenge distorts that pattern of function, the response is to restore the function to that level of normalcy. That is, the cell (tissue, organ, organ system) detects fluctuations and corrects them before the function is altered to a point that puts the cell, tissue, organ, or organism at risk of dying.

At whatever level of study, there are several components necessary for this dynamic equilibrium to develop and to be maintained. There must be a set-point or reference point for each measure. That is, what is the optimal level of function at that biological level (subcellular, cellular, and so on) that maximizes the ability to live and function? This is not a single value, e.g., but a range of values, levels that are compatible with optimal function. This level (with fluctuations) is programmed by the genes. There must be a means of communicating this "information" to an effector, something that is going to bring about a change in function. There has to be a means of getting information back from the effector to the controller to make adjustments in the level of function. This information flow (feed-back) is necessary to keep that function within the limits that determine the normal function of this process—e.g., cell, tissue, organ, organ system. There are age-adjusted clinical values that give guidance about what is considered normal-for-age. Anything outside that range may indicate an impending functional problem. However, it's important to see a larger picture of what's happening with homeostasis—how does it change with aging? What does this mean for the individual? What does this mean when attempting to determine if a function is within or outside what is vital for continued function of the individual? Does homeostatic regulation change due to the aging process? And if there are changes, what are they and how might that impact the function of the older individual? The focus is on the entire individual and the general role that the three system regulators: the nervous system, the endocrine system, and the immune system; play in this change in regulatory function. It can also be done at any of the other biological levels, (subcellular, cellular, tissue, organ, and organ system).

How does an understanding of the change in homeostatic regulation allow one to have a positive impact on the quality of living experience for a person who's older? An overall change is to lessen the severity of the environment—the external physical environment, the psychological environment (both external challenges and internal thoughts and self-perceptions) and the internal environment (e.g., nutrition). Because of the wider range of normalcy, and narrower functional reserve areas, the challenges that alter homeostasis are more "problematic" in the person who is older. The focus should not be on how to correct this wider range of normalcy—the anti-aging focus [34, 35]. Rather it's important to **monitor that function** more carefully, knowing that there is less reserve (or resiliency) and that the challenge may push the person's function over the absolute limit. With this focus, interventions can be undertaken before Ms. A's function exceeds the absolute limits and results in her death.

Clinical Considerations

We don't know what level of genetic or biological reserve (resiliency) Ms. A has. There is no way to definitively say whether she has positive genes, neutral genes, or negative genes. There is nothing (yet) to indicate that her self-neglect is "caused" by her genetics that regulate her biological function. Her outward function is clearly and seriously diminished from what would might be considered "typical" for a person who's 78 years old. One may assume that the negative environmental factors to which she's been exposed throughout her life have interacted with her genetic makeup to heighten her risks of disease and dysfunction. The focus clearly outlined in Part 1 (Key Points) is to address the range of environmental challenges that Ms. A continues to face. The negative environment in which she lives continues to put her at heightened risk of disease or even of early death. These many actions and possible interactions have the goal of helping Ms. A's function remain within her range of normalcy…not to go into the lessened reserve areas. The lessened biological reserve can also be expressed as a decrease in the resiliency of the individual. That is, the lessened ability to "bounce-back" from an environmental challenge before that challenge becomes overwhelming. Effectively using the variety of environmental interventions (which include the medical) can lessen the likelihood that the function in one or more of Ms. A's biological systems will exceed the absolute limit and result in her death.

Key Points

1. Take a complete and thorough social history including a trauma history as this may help in understanding the effect of a negative environment on the subsequent development of self-neglecting behavior.
2. Increase social and family network to benefit the older adult.
3. Assess any community and mental health services that might go into the home
4. More research is needed in order to clearly characterize and diagnose self-neglect so that we can apply consistent treatment modalities.

References

Part I

1. Pickens S, Daniel M, Jones EC, Jefferson F. Development of a conceptual framework for severe self-neglect (SN) by modifying the CREST model for self-neglect. Front Med. 2021;8:1–15. https://doi.org/10.3389/fmed2021.654627.
2. Abrams RC, Reid MC, Lien C, Pavlou M, Rosen A, Needell N, et al. The Abrams Geriatric Self-Neglect Scale: introduction, validation and psychometric properties. Int J Geriatr Psychiatry. 2018;33:e73–84. https://doi.org/10.1002/gps.4718.
3. National Center on Alder Abuse. Types of abuse. 2016. Available online at: https://ncea.ac1.gov/Suspect-Abuse-Types.aspx#self. Accessed 30 Mar 2024.
4. Dong X, Simon MA, Evans DA. Prevalence of self-neglect across gender, race and socio-economic status: findings from the Chicago Health and Aging Project. Gerontology. 2012;58(3):258–68. https://doi.org/10.1159/000334256.
5. Pavlou MP, Lachs MS. Could self-neglect in older geriatric subjects be a geriatric syndrome? J Am Geriatr Soc. 2006;54(5):831–42. https://doi.org/10.1111/j.1532-5415.2006.0661.x.
6. Dong X, Simon MA, Evans D. Elder self-neglect and hospitalization: findings from the Chicago Health and Aging project. J Am Geriatr Soc. 2012;60:202–9. https://doi.org/10.1111/j.1532-5415.2011.03821x.
7. Dong X, Simon MA, Mendes de Leon CF, Fulmer F, Beck T, et al. Elder self-neglect and mortality risk in a community-dwelling population. JAMA. 2009;302:517–26. https://doi.org/10.1001/jama.20091109.
8. Abrams RC, Lachs M, McAvay G, Keohane DJ, Bruce ML. Predictors of self-neglect in community-dwelling elders. Am J Psychiatry. 2002;159(10):1724–30. https://doi.org/10.1176/appi.ajp.159.10.1724. PMID 12359679.
9. Lien C, Rosen T, Bloeman EM, Abrams RC, Pavlou M, Lachs MS. Narratives of self-neglect: patterns of traumatic and maladaptive behaviors in cognitively intact older adults. J Am Geriatr Soc. 2016;64(11):e195–200. https://doi.org/10.1111/jgs.14524. Epub 2016 Oct14. PMID 27739073.
10. Culberson JW, Ticker RI, Marcus MT, Pickens SL, Dyer CB. Prescription use among self-neglecting elderly. J Addict Nurs. 2011;22(1–2):63–8. https://doi.org/10.3109/10884602.2010.545089.
11. Dong X, Simon MA, Evans D. Prospective study of the elder self-neglect and ED use in a community population. Am J Emerg Med. 2012;30:553–61. https://doi.org/10.1016/j.ajem.2011.02008.
12. Liu P, Delagrammatikas L. Adult Protective Services's role in addressing older and dependent adult abuse in the age of COVID. Front Public Health. 2021;9:659640. https://doi.org/10.3389/fpubh.2021.659640.
13. Diagnostic and statistical manual of mental disorders. 5th ed., text revision. American Psychiatric Association; 2022. https://doi.org/10.1176/appi.books.9780890425787.
14. Dong X. Elder self-neglect: research and practice. Clin Interv Aging. 2017;12:949–54. https://doi.org/10.2147/CIA.S103359.eCollection2017. PMID 28652717 PMCID:PMC472408.
15. Pickens S, Burnett J, Ross MET, Jones E. Meeting the challenges in conducting research in vulnerable older adults with self-neglect-notes from a field team. Front Med. 2023:10. https://doi.org/10.3389/fmed.2023.1114895.
16. Day MR, McCarthy G. Self-neglect: development and evaluation of a self-neglect (SN-37) measurement instrument. Arch Psychiatr Nurs. 2016. Available online at: https://daneshyari.com/article/preview/314817.pdf
17. Kelly PA, Dyer CB, Pavlik VN, Doody R, Jogerst G. Exploring self-neglect in older adults: preliminary findings of the self-neglect severity scale and next steps. J Am Geriatr Soc. 2008;56:S253–60. https://doi.org/10.1111/j.1532-5415.2008.01977x.

18. Kohlman-Thomson L. The Kohlman evaluation of living skills. 3rd ed. Bethesda: American Occupational Therapy Association, Inc.; 1992.
19. Hoarding disorder. In Diagnostic and statistical manual of mental disorders, 5th edition, text revision. American Psychiatric Association; 2022. pp. 277–81. https://doi.org/10.1176/appi.books.9780890425787.
20. Dozier ME, Porter B, Ayers CR. Age of onset and progression of hoarding symptoms in older adults with hoarding disorder. Aging Ment Health. 2016;20(7):736–42. https://doi.org/10.1080/13607863.2015.1033684.
21. Morein-Zamir S, Papmeyer M, Pertusa A, Chamberlain SR, Fineberg NA, Shahakian BJ, et al. The profile of executive function in OCD hoarders and hoarding disorder. Psychiatry Res. 2014;215(3):659–67. https://doi.org/10.1016/j.psychres.2013.12.026.
22. Ayers CR, Pittman JOE, Davidson EJ, Dozier ME, Mayes TL, Almklov E. Predictors of treatment outcome and attrition in adults with hoarding disorder. J Obsessive Compuls Relat Disord. 2018;23:100465. https://doi.org/10.1016/j.jocrd.2019.100465.
23. Bratiotis C, Muroff J, Lin N. Hoarding disorder: development in conceptualization, intervention and evaluation. Focus. 2021; published online 5 Nov 2021. https://doi.org/10.1176/appi.focus.20210016.
24. Davidson EJ, Dozier ME, Pittman JOE, Mayes TL, Blanco BH, et al. Recent advances in research on hoarding. Curr Psychiatry Rep. 2020;21(9):91. https://doi.org/10.1007/s11920-019-1078-0. PMID:31410591 PMCID:PMC7294597.
25. Lee JL, Burnett J, Xia R, Smith SM, Dyer CB. Feasibility of intervention in elder self-neglecters: setting the stage for future research. J Elder Abuse Negl. 2018;30:223–35. https://doi.org/10.1080/08946566.20181450172.
26. Liu P, Hass Z, Stratton S, Conrad K, Conrad K. Self-neglect of older adults: how can adult protective services help? Innov Aging. 2022;6:47. https://doi.org/10.1093/geroni/igac059.1601.
27. Hang M, Yuhang W, Xiaojun L, Xiaofan Y, Ping H. Childhood environmental unpredictability and hoarding: mediating roles of attachment and security. Acta Psychol. 2024;244:104–98.
28. Bauman SL. Defiance or self-neglect. Nurs Sci Q. 2023;36(4):346–54. https://doi.org/10.1177/08943184231118786.
29. Burnett J, Hoyumpa G, Kotwal A, Ayieko S, Perissinotto C. Innov Aging. 2023;7(Supplement_1):847–48. https://doi.org/10.1093/geroni/igad104.2732.
30. Dyer CB, Pickens S, Burnett J. Vulnerable elders when it is no longer safe to live alone. JAMA. 2007;298:1448–50. https://doi.org/10.1001/jama.298.121448.
31. Abrams RC, Ansell P, Breckman R, Karlawish J, Lachs M, Holt-Knight D, et al. The interview for decisional abilities (IDA): a tool to assess the decisional capacity of abused and neglected older adults. Elder Abuse Negl. 2019;31(3):244–54. https://doi.org/10.1080/08946566.2019.1573392. Epub 2019 Feb 27.

Part 2

32. Ahmadlou M, Shirazi MY, Zhang P, et al. A subcortical switchboard for perseverative, exploratory and disengaged states. Nature. 2025;639(8053):1–11. https://doi.org/10.1038/s41586-025-08672-1.
33. Farsetti A, Illi B, Gaetano C. How epigenetics impacts on human disease. Eur J Intern Med. 2023;114:15–22. https://doi.org/10.1016/j.ejim.2023.05.036.
34. Doctrow, B. Research in context: can we slow aging? NIH Research Matters 15 Oct 2024. https://www.nih.gov/news-events/nih-research-matters/research-context-can-we-slow-aging
35. Anti-Aging Movement Wikipedia. https://en.wikipedia.org/wiki/Anti-aging_movement
36. Rowe JW, Kahn RL. Human aging: usual and successful. Science. 1987;237(4811):143–9. https://doi.org/10.10.1126/science.3299702

37. Rowe JW, Kahn RL. Successful aging. Gerontologist. 1997;37(4):433–40. https://doi.org/10.1093/geront/37.4.433.
38. The Editors of the Encyclopedia Britannica, Updated: Feb 5, 2025 Homeostasis Physiology. https://www.britannica.com/science/homeostasis
39. Libretti S, Puckett Y. Physiology, homeostasis. [Updated 2023 May 1]. In: StatPearls [Internet]. Treasure Island (FL): StatPearls Publishing; 2025 Jan-. Available from: https://www.ncbi.nlm.nih.gov/books/NBK559138/

Chapter 9
Institutional Abuse and Neglect

Lisa Rachmuth, Jacqueline S. Gray, Veronica LoFaso, and Geoffrey Rogers

Introduction

The growing crisis of elder abuse in institutions demands immediate attention and coordinated response from human services professionals. The National Center on Elder Abuse [29] conducted a nationwide study of elder abuse based on a survey of Adult Protective Services (APS) administrators who provided state-level data on reports of elder and vulnerable adult abuse. Thirteen state APS programs had authority to investigate elder abuse in long-term care settings and reported 6.2% of all substantiated cases of abuse occurred in these settings, while 1.8% occurred in assisted living facilities (and either workplaces or motels/hotels).

As our aging population continues to expand (Urban Institute, 2025; [31]), the complexity and scope of elder abuse cases have evolved, requiring sophisticated understanding and intervention strategies. In this chapter, guidance for medical, legal, social, and human services professionals will include essential knowledge and practical frameworks for addressing institutional elder abuse.

L. Rachmuth (✉)
Division of Geriatrics and Palliative Medicine, Center for Elder Abuse Solutions, Weill Cornell Medicine, New York, NY, USA
e-mail: Lir2034@med.cornell.edu

J. S. Gray
The Native Center for Behavioral Health, University of Iowa College of Public Health, Iowa City, IA, USA

V. LoFaso (Retired)
Division of Geriatrics and Palliative Medicine, Weill Cornell Medicine, New York, NY, USA

G. Rogers
The Learning and Development Projects at the Silberman School of Social Work, Hunter College, City University of New York, New York, NY, USA

V. LoFaso, L. Rachmuth (eds.), *Elder Abuse and Neglect*,
https://doi.org/10.1007/978-3-031-97784-8_9

Definition of Institutional Abuse of Older Adults

How is elder abuse understood? Elder abuse is a single act or repeated acts, or lack of appropriate action, occurring within any relationship where there is an expectation of trust, which causes harm or psychological distress to an older person. Elder mistreatment encompasses neglect as well as physical, psychological/emotional, sexual, and financial abuse. Isolation raises the risk of mistreatment. Multiple factors raise the risk for elder abuse (e.g., poor health, cognitive impairment, functional impairment, low income, low social support, mental illness, substance use, and family violence/trauma). Detection of abuse is hindered when older adults are socially isolated or socially disconnected from their support systems.

Institutional elder abuse is the mistreatment, neglect, and/or exploitation of older adults that occurs in residential facilities or care institutions, such as nursing homes, assisted living facilities, hospitals and group homes. This type of abuse can be committed by staff members, administrators, or other residents, and may include: physical abuse, emotional abuse, neglect, sexual abuse, financial exploitation or ignoring the older person's autonomy. Institutional elder abuse is especially harmful because it often affects vulnerable individuals who rely on the facility for safety and care, and who may have limited ability to report or escape the situation.

Case Presentations

Case 1

Jenny is an 82-year-old white cisgender lesbian female who was brought into the emergency department from her nursing home for leg pain, resulting in constant screaming and cries for help. She was reported to be non-ambulatory in the nursing home but had been ambulatory upon admission one year prior. Jenny was admitted to the nursing home after having lived alone in her apartment with home health care for four hours per day, five days per week. She entered the nursing home after having fallen in her apartment and displaying signs of moderate dementia. She had no relatives or friends who were able to support her. The reason for her admission to the nursing home was based on the inability to support her needs at home, and her rapidly declining cognitive and decisional ability.

Upon examination and x-ray in the emergency department, ED, it was discovered that Jenny had a femur fracture that was at the beginning stages of healing, a stage 3 pressure injury of the sacrum (reportedly being cared for daily at the nursing home), and an extensive fungal infection of the groin. The ED examination concluded that wound care and treatment for the fungal infection and broken femur had not occurred. The reason for the fall was unexplained by Jenny and the nursing home staff contacted upon admission to the ED. The report received by the emergency medical services indicated that the nursing home had been providing regular wound care for the pressure injury. There was no report of any falls or fungal infection.

Case 2

Jerry is a 75-year-old American Indian cisgender male living in a Senior Housing Apartment that was new and unfamiliar to him. Prior to Jerry moving into his current apartment, he was living in his house on the Indian reservation where he grew up. Jerry came into the emergency department by ambulance and was accompanied by his friend Bob. Jerry visited the local senior center daily for meals and conversation with friends. Jerry did not have any other known social connections outside of the senior center. Jerry lived alone and would not accept any visitors to his home. He was a very private person regarding his house and his family relations but was always engaged in conversations with friends. Bob was concerned about Jerry because he had not seen him at the senior center for 2 days; when Bob went to Jerry's house to check on him, Jerry did not respond to Bob's knocks on the door. Bob found that Jerry's door was unlocked and discovered Jerry unconscious on the floor. The house was very cold, and it appeared that Jerry was physically frozen to the floor. EMS were called and were able to separate Jerry from the floor and transported Jerry to the local hospital, where he began to receive care for hypothermia and dehydration. During Jerry's recovery he developed abdominal pain and severe constipation and rectal bleeding. Abdominal x-rays revealed a large amount of stool in the colon. Despite multiple attempts with medications to relieve the constipation, the medical team felt that a rectal examination was needed to disimpact Jerry. During the first conversation about this, he refused. The following day, the medical team again talked to Jerry about the need for the exam and he refused again seemingly without reason. The medical team noted that Jerry's ability to make decisions was not always fluid and rational. Jerry was mostly oriented to place but mixed up the year and where he currently lived. The team assumed he lacked decisional ability though no formal evaluation of his cognitive status or decisional ability was done. Bob was not aware of any family and would not take the responsibility to make medical decisions on Jerry's behalf. The medical team felt it was necessary to proceed with an exam to alleviate the constipation and evaluate for the source of bleeding. They did so without Jerry's consent In the absence of anyone who could advocate for Jerry and under the assumption he lacked decisional ability. They felt they were acting on his behalf. After deep investigation, the hospital social worker was able to locate Jerry's daughter, who had been trying to locate him for weeks. When she arrived to see Jerry and speak with the medical staff, she shared historical information with the medical staff about Jerry's early life on the reservation and at an Indian boarding school. She disclosed the sexual abuse Jerry suffered while at the school. The medical team very quickly realized the traumatization that the examination had caused Jerry.

Institutional Abuse Overview

Understanding the Institutional Landscape

Definition of Institution—An institution is an organization, practice, or relationship in a society to benefit or meet the needs of individuals or groups. An institution's rules and procedures aim to ensure consistent quality of care and safety. Older adults commonly interact with institutions in long-term care settings when receiving care at nursing homes and rehabilitation facilities. They may interact with other types of institutions, such as financial institutions as well. Although discussions of elder abuse often focus on mistreatment by individual people in the community setting, elder mistreatment can also occur in institutions and can include any of the types of elder abuse.

Elder Abuse in the Context of an Institution

Elder abuse in institutions manifests not only through individual actions but also through complex institutional structures that can either protect or harm vulnerable older adults. The institutional framework, which encompasses physical care facilities, healthcare systems, financial institutions, and legal frameworks, plays a crucial role in either preventing or potentially enabling elder abuse.

In institutions, abuse can occur through direct mistreatment or systemic neglect. Inadequate staffing ratios, poor training, and cost-cutting measures often create environments where abuse can flourish unchecked. Healthcare systems may perpetuate harm through discriminatory practices (ex: ageism, sexism or racism), inadequate care protocols, or insufficient attention to the needs of older adults. Financial institutions, despite existing protective measures, may fail to detect, protect, or prevent exploitation of older adults' resources. A 2018 World Health Organization, WHO, report suggests that over 33% of older adults living engaged in institutional settings and over 64% of institution employees reported abuse of older adults [34].

Ageism

Ageism is defined as the systematic stigmatization and discrimination against individuals because of their age. Ageist attitudes and policies often normalize or render invisible the experiences of older people who may be facing abuse [10, 19].

The norms of our culture either revere the aging process or fight the aging process and work to reverse its course. American society is deeply embedded in enhancing youth and rejecting aging [33]. Societal norms dictate and put emphasis on youth and a youthful perspective. We are socialized to understanding aging from a deficit perspective. This prejudice is similar to the prejudice that experience by people inaffecting Black, older and LGBTQ communities. Socio-cultural-political norming of the perceived deficit of minoritized populations in turn normalizes abusing and financial exploitation of older people. Older adults are not understood as an equal partner in our frayed social contract. We understand the older person's humanity as having less value that of the young. This opens the door to the abuse and financial exploitation of older people. Ageism, is correlative of elder abuse [18, 32]. An example of this is that an older adult's historical perspective may not be considered. There are links between ageism, racism, gender bias, and sexual preference bias. Ageist attitudes permeate institutional practices, leading to discriminatory policies and inadequate resource allocation for older people. If aging and older people are valued, we would be more inclined to protect them. When older adults are seen as less valuable it creates a societal framework in which they are more likely to be ignored, targeted and abused. The harmful effects of ageism contribute to the perpetuation of elder abuse, making it harder for victims to be heard or helped or protected [5, 21, 23].

Dementiaism is yet another form of bias that is pervasive in institutions. We know that close to 50% of demented patients experience some form of abuse or neglect. Commonly, this manifests as an older adult reporting abuse or neglect and not being believed leading to serious negative health outcomes.

Red Flags: Identification

Effective identification of elder abuse begins with recognition of abuse indicators. Service professionals must be deliberate about gaining expertise in engagement, and identificating various forms of abuse, from obvious physical harm to subtle psychological manipulation. Medical professional, social service providers, and legal professionals receive limited training and education specific to understanding and identificating elder abuse. Physical abuse may present through unexplained injuries, while psychological abuse often manifests in behavioral changes or withdrawal. Financial exploitation might be revealed through unusual account activity or sudden changes in financial arrangements. This assessment requires a multidisciplinary approach.

Warning signs often extend beyond anecdotal cases to institutional patterns and practices. High staff turnover, persistent morale issues, or patterns of similar complaints across multiple residents residing in an institution may indicate systemic problems requiring broader intervention. Institutional resistance to inquiry or lack of transparency should raise immediate concerns. [20].

Risk assessment matrices may help identify cases and allocate resources effectively. Each case of suspected abuse requires a thorough review including medical, nursing, and administrative practices. Comprehensive evaluation frameworks ensure that no aspect of a case is overlooked. When necessary, safety planning protocols guide immediate intervention strategies [1, 11].

Case Discussion-Case 1

This case highlights several areas where medical, nursing, and administrative services fell short of the expected standard of care resulting an emergency hospitatlization.

The Emergency Room

The ED team noted several red flags for neglect: extensive fungal infection indicating poor hygiene, unexplained femur fracture in a non-ambulatory patient, and a large pressure ulcer with evidence of infection. Although any one of these findings can occur in older adults without there being neglect, the constellation of all three certainly raises concerns and the need for further investigation. The ED team, after having contacted the nursing home to obtain further medical information found the explanation of medical findings inadequate. At that point the social work team would intervene and consideration about whether the patient should be returned to that facility would need to be discussed. Given that she has no family or designated caregiver and lacks decisional ability, proceeding with a guardian may be indicated to advocate for her. A report to APS and state nursing oversight agencies should be made about the negligent care the patient received.

The Nursing Home

Administration

In the case of any fall or injury in a nursing facility, an incident report should be made, the physician should be notified, and the family made aware.

Nursing

There are several areas that call into question the nursing care given in the facility. First, the presence of a large poorly treated pressure ulcer always is of concern. Although pressure ulcers are not always the result of neglect, the severity and poorly cared for wound raises a red flag for neglect. Older individuals with multiple medical conditions who are immobile are at risk and in some cases the pressure ulcers are unavoidable. Many nursing homes use scales to assess the risk of skin breakdown upon admission which determines who is at risk and what the best skin monitoring plan should be. Was this done? Additionally, nursing homes have wound care nurses who specialize in preventing and caring for pressure ulcers. The observation by the ED team of an extensive fungal rash is also of concern and could be a clue to the development of the pressure ulcer. The fact that it was not noted in nursing notes is suspicious for suboptimal care and neglect. The nursing staff should be inspecting the patient's skin with routine hygiene care and alerting the facility physician if any rashes are noted. Ideally this patient would have received frequent personal hygiene care, treatment of the fungal infection and frequent positioning in bed to avoid pressure ulcers. Additionally, a proper mattress, pressure reducing cushions, and an appropriate bed to position the patient would be indicated. The wound care team could have been called in to monitor and treat her pressure ulcer. This care was not documented.

The patient sustained a fracture yet was non ambulatory. Investigation into whether proper falls precautions were taken with the patient should be determined. It has been noted that older adults with severe osteoporosis can have spontaneous fractures without significant force. The fact that the fracture was already showing some healing and that the patient was described as constantly screaming speaks to her being left unattended for some time and experiencing significant pain and distress. The fracture likely occurred days if not weeks before she was taken to the ED. Was she neglected because of her cognitive impairment and her pain was not believed? Was the staff reticent to report the fall for fear of retribution or concerns about the nursing homes status?

Medical

Nursing homes have strict regulations about the frequency of medical examinations of their residents. These examinations should include a review of medications, a physical exam including skin exam, cognitive status exam, and review of any new psychiatric or social issues. In this case it is unclear when the fracture occurred and when/if the physician was notified. Was a thorough skin exam done during the exam? Was pain adequately assessed? Was physical therapy and occupational therapy ordered for her so she could have the proper assistive devices to prevent falls? Was the physician monitoring the status of the pressure ulcer? There should be careful documentation of physical findings on exam and clear orders to ancillary staff about the plan of care.

Intervention: Immediate Response and Long-Term Planning

When abuse is identified, immediate response protocols must be activated swiftly and decisively. Emergency intervention may be necessary to ensure immediate safety, particularly in cases of physical abuse, medication mismanagement, sexual assault, or severe neglect. This might involve emergency medical evaluation, temporary placement in alternative care settings, implementation of crisis management protocols, or interventions involving law enforcement. Professionals should be familiar with their state laws and local protocols related to reporting and handling of elder abuse situations; in most U.S. states, elder abuse falls under mandated reporting laws.

Proving systemic abuse in settings requires clear and precise documentation that is free of bias. Statements of facts is paramount. Evidence preservation becomes crucial, particularly in cases that may require legal intervention. Detailed documentation of injuries, conditions, statements, and circumstances creates a foundation for potential legal proceedings and helps establish repeated patterns of abuse over time [4, 12, 26].

Long-term planning requires careful coordination of multiple services and supports. Comprehensive care plans must address ongoing safety monitoring while coordinating necessary support services. Legal intervention may be required to establish guardianship or protective orders. Financial protection measures might include appointment of financial managers or implementation of fiscal monitoring systems. Financial exploitation is also a devasting and life altering form of abuse [2, 16]. When considering immediate responses or long-term interventions, consideration needs to be given to always identifying and implementing the least restrictive and intrusive form of care, thereby always respecting the older adult's autonomy and right to self-determination. In Jenny's case, could she have been maintained in her home and avoided institutional placement?

Case Discussion-Case 2

Why Is This Institutional Abuse

The right to self-determination should always guide medical care. This tenet assumes that an individual has decisional ability to direct their care even if their decision is at odds with what the medical team feels is best. In this case a formal evaluation of Jerry's decisional ability should have been done. This evaluation would ideally be done by a psychiatrist and would include:

- Did Jerry understand that severe constipation and rectal bleeding can be a sign serious disease such as cancer and can put a person at significant risk
- Did Jerry appreciate that he personally had rectal bleeding and severe constipation causing his pain and putting him at risk for serious health issues
- Could he express the advantages and disadvantages of undergoing the rectal exam? Can he rationally defend his positions?
- Does he consistently make the same choice on repeated questioning

It is important to recognize that individuals with mild cognitive impairment or even early dementia can still make decisions about their health care. Although the medical team felt they were acting on Jerry's behalf they did not properly evaluate Jerry's ability to make decisions. If Jerry's medical situation was critical and psychiatric evaluation of his decisional ability revealed he lacked capacity, then the case should be brought before the Ethics committee of the hospital for review. All attempts should be made to align treatments with Jerry's expressed wishes.

It is of note that the staff did not delve further into why Jerry refused the examination. Although women are more likely to experience sexual abuse, when men are sexually abused they are much less likely to share their experiences. Being alert to non-verbal cues, and unexplained behaviors and decisions is key to uncovering a history of trauma. The medical team might have brought in a psychiatrist or social worker to explore Jerry's resistance and may have been able to work with him to accept the procedure on his terms.

Professionals must have an understanding and skills to address institutional elder abuse effectively. Core competencies include:

- Person centered approaches to assessment, care and treatment
- Trauma-informed care practices ensuring interventions don't create additional harm
- Cultural competency to enable appropriate response to diverse populations
- Knowledge of state laws around elder abuse and elder justice initiatives.

Coordination with legal experts to help navigate laws, complex regulatory frameworks and court systems [3, 15, 17].

Skill development focuses on systems navigation and multi-agency coordination. The complexity of elder abuse cases often requires collaboration across multiple agencies and service providers. Expert testimony skills may be needed for court proceedings. Policy advocacy capabilities help address systemic issues and drive institutional change.

Resource Navigation in Communities

Many municipalities offer a complex network of resources for addressing elder abuse. The servicer providers in these networks may be siloed or coordinated, depending on access to services such as MDTs or coalitions. Emergency services provide immediate response capabilities, while legal aid organizations offer crucial support for court proceedings and protective orders. Healthcare providers specializing in elder care can address medical needs and document evidence of abuse.

Housing assistance becomes crucial when placement changes are necessary [14, 27, 28, 35]. Financial counseling services help address exploitation and establish protective measures. Support groups provide emotional support and connection for isolated older adults. Cultural organizations offer specialized services for diverse communities.

Effective resource utilization requires strong inter-agency partnerships and clear referral protocols. Resource sharing agreements maximize available services while reducing duplication of efforts. Follow-up procedures ensure continuity of care and monitor intervention effectiveness. Outcome tracking helps identify successful strategies and areas needing improvement.

The inability of older adults to navigate community resources can significantly contribute to neglect, impacting their health, safety, and overall well-being. It's crucial to keep in mind the connection between neglect and circumstances arising from poverty, systemic and institutional barriers. The inability to access community resources can significantly contribute to situations that are often experienced as neglect, particularly among families experiencing poverty.

Without access to essential services like healthcare, nutrition programs, and personal care, older adults may experience deteriorating health, malnutrition, and increased risk of injury. This deprivation can be a form of neglect, whether self-imposed due to isolation or resulting from systemic and institutional barriers.

Challenges such as limited mobility, lack of information about available services, and complex procedures can hinder older adults from obtaining necessary support. These obstacles can lead to situations where their needs are unmet, constituting neglect.

Social isolation can exacerbate neglect, as older adults may lack the support network to assist them in accessing resources or recognizing when their needs are not being met. This isolation increases their vulnerability to neglect and other forms of abuse.

To mitigate neglect stemming from inaccessible resources, it's crucial to:

- Invest in infrastructure and policies that prioritize the needs of older adults, ensuring equitable access to essential services.
- Encourage community engagement and support systems to reduce isolation and provide assistance in navigating resources.
- Simplify procedures and improve outreach to ensure older adults are aware of and can easily access available services

By addressing these areas, communities can better support older adults, reducing instances of neglect and promoting healthier, more connected lives.

Documentation and Legal Framework

Proper documentation serves multiple crucial purposes in elder abuse cases. Initial assessments provide baseline information for measuring progress and identifying patterns. Intervention plans outline tactical and strategic approaches and coordinate multiple services. Progress notes track developments and responses to interventions. Incident reports document specific abuse events and response measures. Documentation from various and differing professionals, medical charts, legal documentation, and social work notes all contribute to an accounting of abusive situations.

Understanding the legal framework is essential for effective intervention. State elder abuse laws provide the foundation for protective actions. Mandatory reporting requirements establish clear obligations for professionals who encounter abuse.

Guardianship procedures offer options for protecting vulnerable older adults who cannot advocate for themselves [6].

Privacy regulations must be carefully navigated to protect confidentiality while ensuring necessary information sharing among service providers. Evidence standards guide documentation practices and preparation for potential legal proceedings. Understanding court processes helps professionals navigate legal interventions effectively. Local jurisdictions should be checked for these laws and regulations governing privacy.

Intersectionality and Cultural Respect in Practice

Intersectionality and cultural respect require more than awareness of different traditions, language, and holidays. They demand development of deep cultural knowledge bases and understanding of how cultural factors influence both abuse dynamics and intervention effectiveness. Language access becomes crucial for accurate assessment and effective intervention.

Religious and spiritual sensitivity ensures interventions respect spiritual beliefs and practices. Understanding traditional practices helps distinguish cultural norms from abusive behaviors. Family dynamics often play crucial roles in both abuse patterns and intervention possibilities.

Implementation of cultural respect requires practical measures. Culturally appropriate services must be designed and delivered in ways that respect diverse traditions. Language assistance ensures accurate communication and understanding. Community partnerships provide cultural expertise and connection to relevant resources [9, 25]. Obtaining and reading psychosocial assessments and listening to the patient's experience, gives the professional critical information about their abuse history and their current victimization. Storytelling is a critical tool that can be used [7, 22]. In the previous case scenario, asking the patient to recall (or relate) their negative or positive experience with a previous situation that might be correlated to the current situation.

At age five, Jerry was taken from his parents and placed in a residential boarding school hundreds of miles from his home. This was done without his parents' consent and for no reasons related to child abuse, neglect, or maltreatment. This was a standard protocol done to American Indian/Alaskan Native children starting in the 1870s and ending in the 1960s. The policy behind this was based on Pratt's teachings around the philosophy "Kill the Indian in him and save the man" [24]. Many of the American Indian/Alaskan Native children sent to the boarding schools were abused, neglected, and died from diseases during their time away from their parents. Clothing, hair, diet, practices, language, ceremony, and spirituality were all to be removed from the children so they would be void of their native culture, beliefs, and identity and replaced with "Western Christian" culture, beliefs, values, and practices. While in the boarding school, Jerry was repeatedly sexually abused anally with a broom handle by multiple abusers, both male and female [30]. Knowledge of Jerry's abuse history might have prevented him from being re-traumatized.

Prevention Through Education and Training

Prevention and education form critical components of a comprehensive response to elder abuse. Community education programs must target multiple audiences, including older adults themselves, family caregivers, service providers, community organizations, financial institutions, and healthcare facilities. Professional training must remain current with emerging trends, legal updates, and technological advances while maintaining focus on fundamental skills in communication and ethics.

Prevention efforts must target varied audiences with tailored education programs. Older adults need information about rights, resources, and warning signs. Family caregivers require training in proper care techniques and stress management. Service providers need ongoing education about best practices and emerging trends.

Community-based organizations play crucial roles in prevention through outreach and education. Financial institutions require training to identify and prevent exploitation. Healthcare facilities need protocols for abuse screening and reporting. Courts and legal settings need training in elder law and appropriate ways to address abuse within systems.

Professional development must evolve to address emerging challenges. Best practices continue to develop as understanding of elder abuse grows. Technology creates new risks of exploitation but also provided tools for prevention and intervention. Engagement skills are crucial for effective intervention and support.

Building Collaborative Response Networks

Effective response to elder abuse requires strong collaborative networks. Law enforcement partners provide crucial support in criminal cases. Healthcare providers offer medical expertise and documentation. Legal services navigate complex court proceedings. Financial institutions implement protective measures against exploitation.

Coordination protocols establish clear communication channels and response procedures. Effective strategies for collaboration between disciplines include information sharing agreements that protect privacy, joint investigations, and case conferences, which maximize resources and expertise while enabling planning and intervention.

Quality review processes help identify which strategies have proven effective and highlight areas in need of improvement. Regular evaluation of the success of these collaborative efforts ensures effective resource utilization and optimal outcomes for older adults.

Supporting Professional Health and Excellence

The demanding nature of elder abuse intervention requires strong professional support systems. Stress management becomes crucial for maintaining effectiveness and preventing burnout. Work life balance ensures professionals can give appropriate attention to complex cases [8, 13]. Professional boundaries protect both workers and the older people that they serve.

Support networks provide crucial emotional and practical assistance. Wellness practices help maintain professional resilience. Continuing education ensures skills remain current and effective.

Organizational support must include strong supervision protocols and peer support systems. Professional development opportunities help build necessary skills and knowledge. Resource allocation must prioritize both client services and professional support. Policy advocacy addresses systemic barriers to effective intervention.

Key Points

1. Success demands maintenance of high professional standards while advocating for systemic change. Through coordinated effort, careful documentation, and continuous improvement, the professional community can work effectively to protect older adults and prevent abuse.
2. Financial literacy becomes increasingly important as financial exploitation grows more sophisticated. Risk assessment skills enable proper case prioritization and allocation. Documentation skills ensure proper record-keeping for both case management and potential legal proceedings.
3. Building communities with older adults as an integral part of the eco-system is one way to create a continuum of care. Concerned persons in the lives of older adults can often be the first to identify that an older adult is experiencing elder abuse in an institutional setting; aspire to build intergenerational communities.
4. Training should have a multidisciplinary focus in: aging, ageism, dementiaism, elder abuse, intimate partner violence, legal resources, support, training in specific areas of expertise, cultural respect and acknowledgement of differences, and trauma informed care.
5. Professionals have vital roles in preventing or safeguarding older people from institutional abuse.
6. Social Workers/Human Services professionals can provide detailed assessments of the older adult's history, including previous trauma. Trusted individuals who understand the wishes of the older adult can contribute to the assessment process.
7. Civil Legal Attorneys/District Attorneys have a key role in identifying and assisting the older adult with leaving an abusive institutional setting(s); particularly if the older adult is under guardianship. Monitoring the guardianship is also the role of the courts. Placement issues should be carefully considered by guardians and the courts. Lawyers advocating for the best interest of the older adult in all situations is paramount.

8. Medical Professionals are often the first eyes on an older adult who is abused.
9. Recognizing the indicators of abuse is the first step to helping an older person who is being abused. You do not need to necessarily diagnose abuse definitively. Considering whether the clinical presentation matches the medical situation — i.e., Is this story plausible? Is this framing, similar to other parts of the medical diagnosis? One reason elder abuse, especially neglect, can be difficult to detect is that it can mimic many of the changes of normal aging. The distinctions can be difficult.
10. All professionals can interact with multidisciplinary professional team members. In many states medical, social work, and legal professionals are mandated reporters for elder abuse, but support is needed. Teams within and outside of your facility are often essential in being able to support the older adult to eliminate abuse from their life. Identifying patterns is often something that can be identified once a team of professionals is involved in all cases. If an elder abuse team is available, utilization can only help diminish risk to vulnerable older adults.

References

1. Ageing Equal. Ageism and abuse. 2018. https://ageing-equal.org/ageism-and-abuse/
2. American Psychological Association. 2012. https://www.apa.org/topics/aging-older-adults/elder-abuse.pdf
3. Bergeron LR. Self-determination and elder abuse do we know enough? J Gerontol Soc Work. 2006;46(3–4):81–102. https://doi.org/10.1300/J083v46n03_05. PMID: 16803778. https://pubmed.ncbi.nlm.nih.gov/16803778/
4. Branco IM, Pires L, Afonso RM, Ferreira SFS. Institutional Ageism Perception in Health Contexts Scale (IAPHe): Psychometric study with professionals who work with older adults. Educ Gerontol. 2024; 1–14. https://doi.org/10.1080/03601277.2024.2433269. https://www.tandfonline.com/doi/full/10.1080/03601277.2024.2433269?src=exp-la
5. Combating Abuse. Weill Cornell Medicine. 2025. https://elderabuse.weill.cornell.edu/programs/combating-ageism
6. DOJ. 2022. https://www.justice.gov/elderjustice/prosecutors/statutes
7. Dyer C, Heisler C, Hill C, Kim L. Community approaches to elder abuse. 2005. Clin Geriatr Med. 2005;21(2):429–47. https://www.geriatric.theclinics.com/article/S0749-0690(04)00127-2/abstract
8. Enguidanos S, DeLiema M, Aguilar I, Lambrinos J, Wilber K. Multicultural voices: attitudes of older adults in the United States about elder mistreatment. Ageing Soc. 2014;34(5):877–903. https://doi.org/10.1017/S0144686X12001389. https://pmc.ncbi.nlm.nih.gov/articles/PMC4215730/
9. Friedman and Ranzenhofer. Understanding the New York Elder Abuse Prevention Act. 2025. https://www.wny-lawyers.com/2023/07/understanding-the-new-york-elder-abuse-prevention-act/
10. Hawes C. Elder abuse in residential long-term care settings: what is known and what information is needed? In: National Research Council (US) Panel to Review Risk and Prevalence of Elder Abuse and Neglect; Bonnie RJ, Wallace RB, editors. Elder mistreatment: abuse, neglect, and exploitation in an aging America. Washington (DC): National Academies Press (US); 2003; 14. Available from: https://www.ncbi.nlm.nih.gov/books/NBK98786/

11. Halpern J. 2020. Ageism: the path to elder abuse. My Elder. https://myelder.com/ageism-the-path-to-elder-abuse/
12. Hoover R, Polson M. Detecting elder abuse and neglect: assessment and intervention. Am Fam Physician. 2014;89(6):453–60. https://www.aafp.org/pubs/afp/issues/2014/0315/p453.html
13. Kaindl K. Cross-cultural perspectives on elder abuse and neglect, vol. 4. Centre Interfacultaire de Gerontologie; 2009. https://cigev.unige.ch/files/1915/3976/3817/questionsdage4.pdf
14. Keilitz S, Uekert B, Jones T. Court guide to effective collaboration on elder abuse. National Center for State Courts; 2008. https://bja.ojp.gov/sites/g/files/xyckuh186/files/Publications/NCSC-Court-Guide-to-Effective-Collaboration-on-Elder-Abuse.pdf
15. Keystone Elder Law. Self-neglect: elder abuse or individual choice? 2025. https://keystoneelderlaw.com/self-neglect-elder-abuse-or-individual-choice/
16. Kurrle S, Sadler P, Cameron I. Patterns of elder abuse. J Australia. 1992;157(10):673–6. https://doi.org/10.5694/j.1326-5377.1992.tb137434.x. https://onlinelibrary.wiley.com/doi/abs/10.5694/j.1326-5377.1992.tb137434.x
17. Lagrotteria D. Respecting a person's right to self-determination and autonomy in elder protective services. 2023. https://lifepathma.org/stories/respecting-a-persons-right-to-self-determination-and-autonomy-in-elder-protective-services/
18. MorrisonS..Don'tcallme"old":avoidingageismwhenwritingaboutaging.2023.https://www.nia.nih.gov/research/blog/2023/12/dont-call-me-old-avoiding-ageism-when-writing-about-aging
19. National Institute on Aging. Long-term care facilities: assisted living, nursing homes and other residential care. 2023, October. https://www.nia.nih.gov/health/assisted-living-and-nursing-homes/long-term-care-facilities-assisted-living-nursing-homes
20. NY STATE. 2024. https://ag.ny.gov/press-release/2024/attorney-general-james-secures-45-million-and-delivers-major-reforms-four#:~:text=NEW%20YORK%20%E2%80%93%20New%20York%20Attorney,and%20address%20years%20of%20resident
21. Pelham V. Confronting ageism in healthcare. Cedars-Sinai Blog. 2023. https://www.cedars-sinai.org/blog/confronting-ageism-in-healthcare.html
22. Pickering C, Maxwell CD, Tatro R, Fales K, Hogoboom B. Development and implementation of a coordinated community response to address elder abuse and neglect. J Foren Nurs. 2022;18(3):156–63. https://doi.org/10.1097/JFN.0000000000000378. https://journals.lww.com/forensicnursing/abstract/2022/09000/development_and_implementation_of_a_coordinated.5.aspx
23. Pillemer K, Burnes D, MacNeil A. Investigating the connection between ageism and elder mistreatment. Nat Aging. 2021;1:2. https://doi.org/10.1038/s43587-021-00032-8. https://pmc.ncbi.nlm.nih.gov/articles/PMC10687725/
24. Pratt R. The advantages of mingling Indians with Whites. National Conference of Charities and Correction at the Nineteenth Annual Session Held in Denver, Colorado. Press of Geo H. Ellis. 1882. https://carlisleindian.dickinson.edu/sites/default/files/docs-resources/CIS-Resources_1892-PrattSpeech.pdf
25. Retraining Orders: Orders of Protection for the Elderly. National Network to End Domestic Violence Women's Law. 2024. https://www.womenslaw.org/laws/pr/restraining-orders/orders-protection-elderly/what-order-protection-elderly#:~:text=An%20order%20of%20protection%20for%20the%20elderly%20is%20an%20order,abuse%20against%20an%20elderly%20person.&text=An%20elderly%20person%20is%20considered%20someone%20aged%2060%20or%20older
26. Sengstock M, McFarland M, Hwalek M. Identification of elder abuse in institutional settings: required changes in existing protocols. J Elder Abuse Neglect. 1990;2(1–2):31–50. https://www.ojp.gov/ncjrs/virtual-library/abstracts/identification-elder-abuse-institutional-settings-required-changes
27. Stiegel L. Legal issues related to elder abuse: a pocket guide for law enforcement. American Bar Association: Commission on Law and Aging. 2014. https://bja.ojp.gov/sites/g/files/xyckuh186/files/Publications/ABA-ElderAbuseGuide.pdf

28. Teaster P, Hall J. Elder abuse and the public health. Springer Publishing; 2018. https://www.springerpub.com/elder-abuse-and-the-public-s-health-9780826171320.html?srsltid=AfmBOopFBjGGws-IgKnOxJXTLGBY4apdmmYfbpk0nNrvbrCNUQ0eX_Su
29. Teaster P, Otto J. The 2004 Survey of adult protective services: abuse of adults 60 years of age and older. (February 2006). The National center on elder abuse. 2006.
30. Upstander Project. 2025. https://upstanderproject.org/learn/guides-and-resources/first-light/pratts-speech
31. Urban Institute. US population is aging. 2025. https://www.urban.org/policy-centers/cross-center-initiatives/program-retirement-policy/projects/data-warehouse/what-future-holds/us-population-aging
32. Weir K. Ageism is one of the last socially acceptable prejudices. Psychologists are working to change that, vol. 54. American Psychological Association; 2023. p. 2. https://www.apa.org/monitor/2023/03/cover-new-concept-of-aging
33. World Health Organization. Ageing: ageism. 2021, March 18. https://www.who.int/news-room/questions-and-answers/item/ageing-ageism
34. WHO, Yon Y, Ramiro-Gonzalez M, Mikton CR, Huber M, Sethi D. The prevalence of elder abuse in institutional settings: a systematic review and meta-analysis. Eur J Public Health. 2018;29(1):58–67. https://doi.org/10.1093/eurpub/cky093. World Health Organization, 2018.
35. Yan E, To L, Wan D, Xie X, Wong F, Shum D. Strategies to build more effective interventions for elder abuse: a focus group study of nursing and social work professionals in Hong Kong. BMC Geriatr. 2022;22(1):978. https://doi.org/10.1186/s12877-022-03682-4. PMID: 36536315; PMCID: PMC9762662. https://pmc.ncbi.nlm.nih.gov/articles/PMC9762662/

Suggested Reading

Brandon P. Caregiver stress can lead to elder abuse. Ageucate Training Institute; 2025. https://blog.ageucate.com/caregiver-stress-can-lead-to-elder-abuse

Caplan Z. U.S. older population grew from 2010 to 2020 at fastest rate since 1880 to 1890. United States Census Bureau. 2023, May 25. https://www.census.gov/library/stories/2023/05/2020-census-united-states-older-population-grew.html

Klodawsky, H. Stolen Times. Documentary Film. 2023.

Lachs MS, Pillemer KA. Elder abuse. Lancet. 2004;364(9441):1263–72. https://doi.org/10.1016/S0140-6736(04)17144-4.

Merriam-Webster. 2025. https://www.merriam-webster.com/dictionary/institution

Mitchell N.. Tips on maintaining professional boundaries for caregivers. Care Academy. 2025. https://careacademy.com/blog/tips-on-maintaining-professional-boundaries-for-caregivers/

Spiritual Abuse article: Gray JS. LaBore KB, Carter P. Protecting the sacred tree: conceptualizing spiritual abuse against Native American elders. Psychol Relig Spirit. Advance online publication. 2018, June 25. https://doi.org/10.1037/rel0000195.

Taylor T. Occupational stress of adult protective service workers. Walden Dissertations and Doctoral Studies. 11860. 2023. https://scholarworks.waldenu.edu/dissertations/11860

World Health Organization. Abuse of older adults. 2024, June 15. https://www.who.int/news-room/fact-sheets/detail/abuse-of-older-people#:~:text=Key%20facts,are%20experiencing%20rapidly%20ageing%20populations

Yon Y, Mikton CR, Gassoumis ZD, Wilber KH. Elder abuse prevalence in institutional settings: a systematic review and meta-analysis. Eur J Pub Health. 2017;27(1):101–7. https://doi.org/10.1093/eurpub/ckw123.

Chapter 10
Undue Influence

Arlene Markarian and Nancy Needell

Introduction

Undue influence is a subtle but nonetheless devastating form of elder abuse. Individuals who are vulnerable or dependent on others either physically or emotionally, can be manipulated, coerced, deceived, isolated or threatened to act in a way that serves the perpetrator yet is at odds with the victim's best interest or wishes. The basic premise is that there is unequal power in a relationship whereby the victim succumbs to the perpetrator's wishes for fear of losing the perpetrator's emotional, financial or physical support, or love.

Case Presentation

Ms. G is a 78-year-old widowed Caucasian woman who lives with her 46 year-old son, Henry, in a two bedroom house she has owned for over 30 years. Her husband died when Henry was 12 and she raised him as a single mother, working as a lunchroom attendant in the local middle school, which he attended. She also worked evenings as a cleaner at several small businesses in their neighborhood. She retired from her job at the school at age 67 as a result of a mandatory retirement policy.

A. Markarian
Safe Observant Seniors Program, FCA-Family and Children's Center, Garden City, NY, USA

N. Needell (✉)
Psychiatry, Weill Cornell Medicine, New York, NY, USA
e-mail: nneedell@med.cornell.edu

V. LoFaso, L. Rachmuth (eds.), *Elder Abuse and Neglect*,
https://doi.org/10.1007/978-3-031-97784-8_10

She continued the cleaning jobs until she was 74, when her arthritis made it impossible for her to complete her tasks.

Henry dropped out of high school in the 11th grade as the result of "dyslexia and Attention Deficit Disorder, (ADD)" and throughout his life has had trouble maintaining steady employment. He does occasional work as a mover and a food delivery person but spends most of his time "hanging around" the local stores and bars.

Police were called to the home multiple times over the past 2 years for erratic behavior by Henry. EMS was also called on several occasions, and drug and alcohol use was noted on drug testing. Henry repeatedly refused inpatient treatment for mental health or drug related issues.

On those visits to the home, officers noted that Ms. G looked thinner and less well-groomed at each visit and the house, usually exceedingly neat, was messy with dirty dishes in the sink and a smell of garbage. When interviewed, Henry dominated the conversation, stating that police and EMS should "mind their business."

One day, during a snowstorm, the police were called to the house because neighbors saw that the front door was open, and they found Ms. G lying on the floor in just a thin nightgown. The house was freezing cold. Furniture was upended and there was spoiled food on the table and floor. Henry was not home and Ms. G was not able to tell them what happened. She was brought to the hospital and admitted for dehydration and hypothermia. Two days later, Henry came to the hospital and demanded to take his mother home. He said that he was away "on a job" and came home to find her missing. He accused the hospital of holding her "hostage" and the police of breaking into the house. He became extremely agitated. Hospital security was called, resulting in the police being called and attempting to arrest Henry.

Ms. G begs them not to arrest Henry and says that she was not able to care for herself without Henry, explaining that this is why she was in such bad shape when the police came to the house. She calls herself "a silly old woman" and says that her poor condition is proof of what a good son and caretaker Henry is. She asks to go home with him and says that now that he is back, she knows she will be in good hands. The hospital discharges her home with Henry but makes an Adult Protective Services referral.

Two weeks later, APS becomes concerned when they get a call from the local bank, saying that Ms. G and Henry showed up seeking to use her house as collateral for a loan. Ms. G had paid off her mortgage years ago and never missed a payment. She now says that she wants to help Henry start a business, She is convinced that he has taken such good care of her over the years and it is her turn now to take care of him. The bank says they need to look things over and Henry gets enraged and storms out.

Later that night, the police are again called to the house and find Henry standing over Ms. G, berating her. She has red marks on her face and bruises in different stages of healing on her arms. The police arrest Henry over her objections. She tells the police that Henry was frustrated because his business needed the money.

This marks the first time Henry has been arrested for any of the domestic disputes in the home. Ms. G goes to the police station and then to court to ask for charges to be dropped. She says that he is a "very good boy" who has had difficulty because of his ADD and that she has failed him and wants to help him get his feet on the ground in this new business. She begs the judge to let him come home with her because she needs him to take care of her, which is why he has never been able to stick with a job. She apologizes to him in front of the police and the judge and "promises" to be a better mother.

The judge reluctantly agrees to drop the charges. Henry promises to control his temper and be respectful to his mother.

The next day, Ms. G calls a lawyer to try to sign ownership of the house over to Henry so that he can fund his business. The lawyer does a quick assessment of the situation and decides that Ms. G understands the consequences of what she is doing and agrees to assist with this transaction. Henry takes ownership of the house and immediately takes a loan against its value. He does not pay back and loses the money. The police are called to the house at least ten more times for verbal disputes.

The bank begins the process to repossess the house and Ms. G is informed that she and Henry must find a new place to live. That night, the police are again called to the house and find Ms. G bleeding and sobbing on the floor. Henry is asleep at the dining room table, which has several empty pill and alcohol bottles on it. They are both taken to the hospital. Henry is placed under arrest for assault and once she is strong enough, Ms. G again asks the police to drop the charges, claiming it is her fault for not being supportive while Henry's business is struggling. This time, the judge declines her request, and Henry is discharged from the hospital to jail. Upon discharge from the hospital, Ms. G begins trying to sell her jewelry to hire a "good lawyer" for Henry.

Undue Influence Overview

The criteria for undue influence are stated in this definition from the American Bar Association:

Undue influence means excessive persuasion that causes another person to act or refrain from acting by overcoming that person's free will and results in inequity. In determining whether a result was produced by undue influence, all of the following shall be considered:

1. Vulnerability of the victim: Evidence of vulnerability may include, but is not limited to, incapacity, illness disability, injury, age, education, impaired cognitive function, emotional distress, isolation, or dependency where the influencer knew of, or should have known of, the alleged victim's vulnerability.
2. The influencer's apparent authority. Evidence of apparent authority may include but is not limited to, status as a fiduciary, family member, care provider, health care prosessional, legal professional, or spiritual adviser.
3. The actions or tactics used by the influencer: Evidence of actions or tactics used may include, but is not limited to, all of the following:

- Controlling necessities of life, medication, the victim's interactions with others, access to information or sleep.
- Use of affection, intimidation, or coercion.
- Initiation of changes in person or property rights, use of haste or secrecy in effecting those changes, effecting changes at inappropriate time and places, and claims of expertise in effecting change.
- The equity of the result: Evidence of the equity of the result may include, but is not limited to, the economic consequences to the victim, any divergence from the victim's prior intent or course of conduct or dealings, the relationship of the value conveyed to the value of any services or consideration received, or the appropriateness of the change in light of the length and nature of the relationship. Evidence of an inequitable result, without more, is not sufficient to prove undue influence.

In New York State, for example, the law requires that judges and juries consider the aforementioned factors above. The four factors are weighted equally, which means that no factor is more important than another; not all four factors have to be present to identify as undue influence.

There are many instances in which undue influence can play out in terms of older adults, but one of the most disturbing and hard to recognize scenarios is when both parties are related. It is hard for many people to imagine a child taking advantage of their older parent, but this happens more frequently than people realize and the undue influence can be quite subtle. Many times, in fact, people working in the elder abuse field do not always agree that undue influence is occurring, which makes it very difficult to identify and to intervene. [5–7].

Examples of undue influence that do not necessarily involve older adults include a boss demanding sexual favors from a subordinate and threatening to fire them if they do not consent, a physician saying he will not treat a patient unless they agree to enroll in a clinical trial, or a teacher threatening to fail a student unless they write a glowing review of the class.

Case Discussion

Psychiatrist's Perspective

This case describes clear abuse and criminal behavior, complicated by the maternal relationship. Throughout the years, Henry used his relationship with his mother as leverage for her to give him money and comply with his abusive behaviors. Henry has always been able to manipulate his mother and coerce her into doing whatever he asks her to do, while also covering up his physically and psychologically abusive behaviors.

Ms. G was able to live with her son's behavior for many years but as she aged, she was no longer able to work two jobs to support them. Henry was not contributing financially to the household. As Ms. G's needs increased, Henry was not able to meet her care needs. As time went on, Henry became angrier at her for her dependence on him and for her inability to care for and financially support him. Henry used this as a manipulative strategy to influence Ms. G to sign her house over to him.

As visits by the police to their home increased, her guilt and shame increased and his behavior towards her worsened. She became more and more afraid of what would happen to him if she could not provide for him and protect him. He became more emotionally and physically abusive towards her and began making increasingly impossible financial demands on her. In addition, his substance use increased, and he relied upon her to pay for his drug habit.

Ms. G has the right to decide to continue to care for Henry and is making a free decision to let him live in her home and to give him money. This is not undue influence. When he begins to exploit her worries, financially coerce her to finance his business, and finally physically abuses her, he crossed the line to undue influence. She has gone from being scared for him to being scared of him. He is using her vulnerable position to intimidate her into doing what he wants to the detriment of her well-being. [4].

Henry's hold over his mother meets the criteria for undue influence—there is an unequal relationship, he is in a position to abuse his power over her (exploiting her fear that he will come to a bad end), and there is a clear benefit to him (getting to live rent free and have someone pay for his lifestyle). This case shows us that there are times when we must consider more than just the superficial facts and delve deep into the situation.

Henry has had years and years of manipulating and living off of his mother and knows exactly how much she loves him and worries about him. We can imagine that she has tried to "put her foot down" in the past, telling him to get a job and asking him not to drink and use drugs in the house. She surely knows of the dangers faced by people who are addicted to drugs and alcohol and does not want these things for her child. When she has tried in the past to "cut him off," she worries that these fates might befall him. She has allowed him to live rent-free in her home while she worked two jobs because she fears that if she throws him out, he will resort to criminal behavior to get the money for drugs and might get arrested—or worse.

Ms. G, who has loved, cared for, and protected her troubled son all his life, is not likely to be willing to be the cause of her son's homelessness, incarceration, or death, especially if she has the means and ability to prevent these outcomes. So, it is not hard for us, given the manipulation, physical and emotional abuse, to understand why she continues to cover for him time and time again when the neighbors call the police to report yelling and noise. Ms. G is the victim of undue influence.

Opportunities for Intervention

When police began coming to the house regularly, it might have been helpful to involve social, mental health, and legal services, who would have been able to offer mental health and substance abuse treatment options to both Henry and Ms. G. If Ms. G knew that such entities as Mental Health and Drug Treatment courts existed, she might have been more amenable to legal interventions—sometimes, the only way people will accept the help they need is if the alternative is going to jail. It is possible that Henry might have benefitted from some of the alternative to incarceration programs that are being developed around the country to divert people from jail and into care. Another service provided by home-based mental health programs is that of a peer advocate, [3] someone who themselves is a recipient of mental health and/or substance abuse services and who can help guide a person into treatment but reducing stigma and serving as a role model and mentor.

Many people along the way determined that Ms. G. had decision making capacity though a formal capacity evaluation was never done. Assessing capacity in cases of undue influence is very difficult as it involves the basic guiding principle of assuming autonomy in decisional capacity. Put more simply, people have the right to make bad decisions, to make decisions that others might disagree with, and might even go against their own best interests. It is assumed that people retain the right to make their own decisions regardless of the consequences as long as they understand the risks and benefits of making those decisions, even if the outcome is detrimental to themselves. [1] For example, a person has the right to refuse potentially life -saving medical care if they can clearly state that they know they might die if they do not get the care and if they can express clearly and rationally that they feel that the medical intervention might cause them more distress than the risk of dying would. A less dramatic assumption of capacity is a person who wishes to invest all of his money in the stock market, knowing that they may lose it all, but are willing to take this risk because the possibility of a big windfall outweighs their concerns about financial ruin. We do not take away someone's right to get married simply because they pick the wrong partner. It is a central tenet of our society that people have the right to make their own decisions unless they have a clear inability to reason. At what point does a situation like Ms. G's change from making a bad decision to undue influence? It is essential to remember that capacity changes with time and circumstance. At some point along the way, her fears of what might happen to him if she did not meet his demands clouded her judgment to make rational decisions about her own wellbeing. [8–10].

It is important that the issue of decisional ability and capacity be considered on a regular basis when working with older adults who are at risk of being the victims of undue influence. While this case discusses undue influence at the hands of a child who uses his mother's unconditional love for him, there are many other possible avenues of undue influence as well—the home attendant who threatens to withhold needed care, the relative or guardian who threatens to put a person in a nursing home or not allow someone to see their grandchildren, the neighbor who threatens to tell a landlord that a person cannot care for herself. The list of potential ways that a lonely, frail, helpless older person can be the victim of unseen—but very real—undue influence is long and those who work with older adults need to be aware of the concept in order to ensure that the people we are working to protect are not suffering silently due to abuse of authority in unequal power relationships.

Prosecutor's Perspective

The case discussed above is all too familiar to law enforcement and prosecutors: the case of an adult child still dependent emotionally and financially on a parent and a living situation that is fraught with turmoil.

In this case we see escalation of Henry's erratic behavior over time. In addition to dozens of calls to the police, Henry became more emboldened, dismissing neighbors' concerns and dominating conversations with police. He was aware that his mother was protecting him from the police. This manipulative behavior is consistent with perpetrators of undue influence using power and control over their victims. Over time this situation escalated to a dangerous level. Henry has either no fear of how he is acting in public at the hospital and or is unable to control himself.

The fact that Ms G. never missed a mortgage payment and paid off her mortgage is proof that she had good financial habits even during the many years of supporting her son until she couldn't work anymore. At that point things escalated in the household coinciding with increasing police calls to the home. While Henry may not have been abusive to her before, the abuse is now escalating. A prosecutor would want to delve further into what occurred and why.

In the incident where Ms. G was found on the floor, evidence appears to show that there was an argument, Henry was angry, and he may have pushed his mother and he left in a hurry without closing the door behind him. A prosecutor might consult a medical professional as asking why Mrs. G was unable to get up off the floor. Was she dehydrated before the fall? Had she missed taking medication? How long did it take for her to get to the stage of hypothermia? What else does a medical exam reveal? Are there any other injuries to her including blunt trauma to her head or other parts of her body that explain what happened and why she wasn't able to get up off the floor? There are many other questions a prosecutor would want answered depending on the specifics of the case.

This would be a 'must arrest' situation in some states, and would probably be a felony assault charge based on her age [2]. It is important to note, Ms. G didn't deny that Henry physically harmed with her rather she gave an excuse for why he assaulted her. It was evident that he had no remorse.

It is unlikely a judge would dismiss this case at this stage of arraignment. A more likely scenario is that the District Attorney would object to a dismissal. If the Judge did not dismiss the case at the arraignment, the DA could speak with Ms. G in a safe place without the offender present. The DA could explaina all the options including the possibility of Drug Treatment Court or Mental Health Court as a possible plea offer. The DA would decide if they have enough evidence to go forward on the case (with or without Ms. G's testimony). If it is a felony charge, in New York State, they would have 6 months to determine whether the case would move forward. During this time, the DA could extend a plea offer to the defense including treatment in exchange for indicting or going to trial. Additionally, the judge would likely issue a Limited Order of Protection at the arraignment which would have permitted Henry to go back home with Ms. G but ordered him to not harass her or commit any offenses against her. In contrast to a full Order of Protection which would have ordered Henry to completely stay away from his mother. Orders of Protection, (or Restraining Orders in some jurisdictions), can have many types of conditions including prohibiting an offender from being in the presence of the victim while under the influence of alcohol or drugs. [11–13].

In Ms. G's situation she was most likely afraid of her son and afraid he would hurt her again. In the author's experience, once the abuser acts violently to a loved one, the relationship forever changes—the victim can't forget what the abuser did and will always wonder if their abuser will hurt them again. The victim will try not to anger their abuser by avoiding honest exchanges, and always agree with the abuser. In this author's experience, victims describe their relationships with abusers as cautious, and have said it is like 'walking on eggshells'.

Manipulation by an adult child perpetrator can include threats of committing suicide, conjuring up a vision of being raped, beaten or assaulted in jail, or having to live in a shelter. These behaviors are used to influence whether or not the victim will comply with the perpetrator's requests, such as giving them money. This is also evidence of undue influence [14–17].

Prosecutor's Tips

- *Subpoena her medical records* to determine why she didn't get up and how long it would take to get in the condition she was found. Speak with her doctor and explore possible explanations for Ms. G's condition when she was found on the floor
- Create *a timeline* in a case like Ms. G's. The timeline should include every call to the police and the evidence of what happened. Body camera footage of the defendant can show an angry man who is screaming at his mother, calling her names and saying this is all her fault. Police reports and EMS/Medical observations should also be included. This timeline can show how the abuse is escalating, and how despite mom's claims that she is not scared of him, that she, in fact, is. This timeline will also help you organize your evidence so you can analyze your case and properly prepare it for court or legal documents like petitions or motions.
- Obtain Henry's *recorded jail calls* to his mother to ascertain threats. Calls to his attorney would be exempt. Does he call her each day or multiple times per day

harassing her? Is he demanding, threatening on the calls, and then crying and claiming he is being beaten or worse while in jail? Is he yelling, cursing, calling her names and blaming her saying it is all her fault he is in jail? Often one can see how the conversations may start off sweet, begging, crying and then escalate to horrible nasty name calling, threats, and yelling to get Ms. G. to do what they want.

- While Undue Influence itself may not be a crime in some states, evidence of it can be used to prove larceny charges or other crimes, or to show that a victim did not give their money or property to the offender of their own free will. This is where the timeline helps—the history of abuse by the offender is very relevant. It is very important for the interviewer to "peel back the onion" when trying to gather this information. Obtaining documents via the Freedom of Information Act or if there is a civil or criminal investigation, via subpoena for each incident is recommended. The more details gathered the better chance of prosecution. Evidence of undue influence will also be important in civil proceedings including Guardianship, Family Court, Landlord/Tenant, and Foreclosure proceedings.
- Below is a list of examples of the types of evidence this author recommends you look for this list is not exhaustive, just illustrative.

  - 911 calls
  - Recorded jail/prison calls
  - Incident recordings; Courthouse cameras Store cameras; Bank cameras; Cell phone recordings; police body cameras.
  - Anything that shows the abusers behavior towards the victim: Voicemails; social media posts; emails; letters or other writings; police reports; medical records.
  - Photographs of any injuries, any marks or bruises anywhere on body damaged property around the home including sentimental items.
  - Financial records: showing her usual practices, past and present: In this case, always paid bills on time; paid off mortgage and now she is going to lose her home
  - Document your records; medical records, attorney records, social work, etc: dates, times and what was said and by whom; document what your client/victim said and what the alleged abuser said; observations re; demeanor; injuries, etc.
  - Specific incidents/dates are important—make that time-line!!

- The author recommends that you ask your patient/client these questions in a private, safe place without anyone else present. This list is not exhaustive, just illustrative.
  "Has anyone"….
- made you afraid? Including in your family? Or anyone that comes to see you?
- tried to physically harm you?
- tried to scare you or threaten you?

- tried to touch you without your permission in a way that makes you feel uncomfortable?
- called you names or cursed at you?
- made you stay in your room; told you that are sick when you are not?
- forced you to do anything that you don't want to do?
- refused to help you when you needed help?
- stopped you from going out or having visitors or talking on the phone?
- prevented you from going to a doctor or a hospital or refused to take you?
- refused to give you your medications or forced you to take too much?
- taken your cane, walker, hearing aid, dentures, eyeglasses, prosthetic, wheelchair, etc without your permission and refused to give them back?
- controlled your food intake? Locked up food so you don't have access?
- threatened to put you in a nursing home?
- taken your money or possessions without your permission or against your will?
- made you sign documents?
- broken your possessions to scare you?
- threatened to hurt other family members or your pets? Removed your pet against your will?

Key Points

- People with capacity have the right to make what we think are 'bad' decisions—even ones that go against their own best interests.
- Decision making capacity can change with time and circumstance, so it is important to reassess capacity as a person's situation changes.
- Undue influence is not always visible to outsiders; you will not see undue influence unless you specifically look for it. It is not undue influence if a person makes a decision because they are afraid for you and what you might do, but it is undue influence if that decision is made because they are afraid of you and what you might do.
- Never underestimate the intensely powerful love a parent has for their child and the lengths they will go to in order to protect that child from harm. Before we judge an older adult we should consider their autonomy in the decisions they make. Guilt can play a role in the course of action they choose; we should be aware of blaming the victims.
- Utilize a multidisciplinary team approach to understand all the factors of the situation. Medical and social work professionals can help shed light on complex situations. Social workers can assist with questioning and creating a safety plan with the victims.
- It is important to remain unbiased and not make assumptions about what a victim may be feeling or experiencing. Not every victim of abuse is the same or reacts to abuse in the same way and interventions should be tailored to the individual.
- Careful and complete documentation in your records is crucial. Photographs, texts, emails, voicemails left for you, social media posts, and security recordings all help create a coherent story. Documenting date, time, and place of concerning or relevant observations of both the victim and the abuser all are important.

- You must check your state laws concerning Undue Influence of an Older Adult. Undue Influence is not a crime in every state, including New York. However the facts and evidence that give rise to undue influence can be used in some criminal cases to prove crimes such as larceny, neglect, or other crimes.

References

1. Abrams R, et al. The Interview for Decisional Abilities (IDA): a tool to assess the decisional capacity of abused and neglected older adults. J Elder Abuse Neglect. 2019;31(3):244–54.
2. NYS Penal Law section 120.05 (12).
3. Power A, Bartlett R. Peer advocacy in a personalized landscape: the role of peer support in a context of individualized support and austerity. J Intellect Disabil. 2016;20(2):183–93.
4. Quinn MJ. Undoing undo influence. J Elder Abuse Neglect. 2000;12(2):9–17.
5. Wolfson W. Study: financial abuse of older adults by family members more common than scams by strangers. Keck School of Medicine of USC. 2019. https://keck.usc.edu/news/study-financial-abuse-of-older-adults-by-family-members-more-common-than-scams-by-strangers/
6. Katz JD. Challenging a will: a guide to understanding undue influence and elder abuse. 2025. https://jdkatz.com/challenging-a-will-a-guide-to-understanding-undue-influence-and-elder-abuse/
7. Safe Harbor Estate Law. Spotting financial elder abuse in your family: 4 Tell-Tale Signs. 2025. https://safeharborestatelaw.com/financial-exploitation-of-the-elderly-by-family-members/
8. Elder Justice Decision Making Capacity Symposium: The role of decision-making capacity in elder justice cases that reach civil and criminal courts. US Department of Justice. 2022. https://www.justice.gov/d9/fieldable-panel-panes/basic-panes/attachments/2022/08/10/decision_making_capacity_resource_guide_corrected_11.1.22.pdf
9. Department of Justice (DOJ) Video. Assessing cognitive capacity in elder abuse cases. 2017. https://www.justice.gov/elderjustice/video/assessing-cognitive-capacity-elder-abuse-cases
10. Center for Elders and the Courts. Key legal issues. National Center for State Courts. 2025. https://www.eldersandcourts.org/aging/aging-material-for-right-rail-menu-for-aging/key-legal-issues
11. Center for Court Innovation. Elder justice bench guide. NYState Unified Court System and NY State Judicial Committee on Elder Justice. 2016. https://www.nycourts.gov/legacypdfs/EJ-Bench-Guide.pdf
12. FindLaw. New York Consolidated Laws, Penal Law - PEN § 120.05 Assault in the second degree. 2024. https://codes.findlaw.com/ny/penal-law/pen-sect-120-05/
13. Nursing Home Abuse Center Blog. Elder abuse restraining orders. 2020. https://www.nursinghomeabusecenter.com/blog/elder-abuse-restraining-orders/
14. Evans Law. Understanding undue influence in elder financial exploitation cases. 2025. https://www.evanslaw.com/practice-areas/financial-elder-abuse/understanding-undue-influence-in-exploitation-cases/
15. American Bar Association (ABA). Undue Influence and Financial Exploitation. 2020;42(2). https://www.americanbar.org/groups/law_aging/publications/bifocal/vol-42/vol%2D%2D42-issue-2%2D%2Dnovember-december-2020-/undue-influence-and-financial-exploitation/
16. Haber J. First department sustains undue influence and unjust enrichment claims in financial exploitation case. Freiberger Haber LLP. 2023. https://fhnylaw.com/first-department-sustains-undue-influence-and-unjust-enrichment-claims-in-financial-exploitation-case/
17. Rahn S. The ultimate guide to undue influence. 10 RMO. 2024. https://rmolawyers.com/blog/undue-influence-guide/

Suggested Reading

ABA Groups Commission on Law and Aging. Publications Bifocal. 2014;35(3). https://www.americanbar.org/groups/law_aging/

Chapter 11
Voice of a Survivor

Cynthia Amodeo

Interviewer: Cynthia Amedeo

Survivor: PR, Anonymous

Victims of abuse are deeply affected by their experiences and carry the trauma with them throughout their lives. Unfortunately for these individuals the abuse may not be a single event but often only one of repeated traumas they suffer for a lifetime. These events can begin in childhood, carry through to interpersonal violence as adults, and sadly, then continue into later years of life.

The sequelae of this trauma can have psychological, physical, and emotional implications. The potential for poor self-esteem can impair their ability to reach their potential and lead independent, successful, lives, and even result in self-neglect.

Below is an interview by a social work professional with a survivor, PR. PR is a victim of life-long violence.

Interviewer: Tell me about yourself.

PR: I was born and raised in Colombia, the second of seven children. In the early 1990s, I came to New York City, USA, hoping to build a good life for myself and make my mother proud. I am currently retired. I was a graphic designer, architectural drafter, and social events organizer, specializing in the art of airbrushing. I created hand-drawn stencils and applied them to a variety of mediums. My work includes body painting, designing logos for businesses, creating architectural models, and drafting building plans by hand. I previously owned my own business and also worked as an art teacher for adults.

C. Amodeo (✉)
Barrier Free Living, Bronx, NY, USA
e-mail: cynthiaa@bflnyc.org

V. LoFaso, L. Rachmuth (eds.), *Elder Abuse and Neglect*,
https://doi.org/10.1007/978-3-031-97784-8_11

Interviewer: Tell me about your abuse history. Please include: Childhood, Sexual, IPV, DV, Victim of a crime by a stranger, Undue influence, Financial Abuse/ exploitation, psychological abuse, emotional abuse.

PR: I have survived both child abuse and domestic violence. The abuse started when I was 5 years old when I was raped by a stranger. As a teenager, I was an assistant to my father, and one of his best friends asked to teach me how to drive, telling me not to tell anyone. I told my mom about the lessons. In the third class, he started to talk to me about sex. At first, I just thought this was an adult teaching me about life lessons. My parents never spoke to me about any of this. Then he started to tell me that he could teach me a lot of things and started to touch me inappropriately while driving, causing me to nearly crash the car. I felt so scared that I wanted to yell and run away but I couldn't. When I got back home my mother and grandmother were praying. When I tried to tell my mother and grandmother, they did not respond and simply continued praying.

My father was abusive only towards me. We had a different relationship than my other siblings. When we were kids he called all of his daughters his princesses. He was very protective of me as a child and let me set up an art business in his office. My father was my hero until I was 15. My father taught me many things such as how to fix things at home, draw, and be responsible. My father emphasized the importance of learning. He was always buying us books. Like my dad, I learned a lot on my own by reading and observing. He was very intelligent but not emotionally connected. I am more because of him.

However, my mother seemed to dislike me and I was often punished for things I didn't understand. For example, (she)would beat me with my father's belt if I got the wrong item from the store. When I got a little older I learned to hide under the bed or go to the shower to protect myself. One time, my father hit me 31 times with his belt, and my mother told me to cry so he would stop. I got up and started to scream at him that I would not cry no matter how many times he hit me. I later learned that my grandmother gave birth to my father at the age of 14. She was assaulted by a married man who did not recognize my father as his. At the age of 4, my father began to work on the farm to help his mother. It was at the farm when he began to be beaten.

When I was a teenager, my father left my mother for another woman. This caused a rift in our family, and I felt embarrassed. Around this time, I began failing my classes in high school, as I was very hyperactive and had trouble focusing. My father did not speak to me for 2 months, which was worse than any other punishment. It was also at this time that all the kids had to go to work because my dad wasn't giving as much to the household and my mom needed money to make ends meet. Sometimes my dad would come over because my mom said I needed a beating. He would pretend to hit me and I would hide under the covers like it hurt.

I always had a voice. When my father would yell at me I would talk back. For example, when he would say "I will break your teeth if you continue to speak to me that way" I would respond by showing him my teeth and say "Go ahead and break them. Then go give my mom the money to fix them." He tried to control my interactions with my friends and in particular men. I never accepted this and that made my father even more frustrated with me. At one point my father told me I had to get a job because I went to a party and did not go home on time. He said he would only pay for food and shelter. I found a job at a local clothing store. One day a man approached me to smuggle goods from the store to another country and get into prostitution. I ended up quitting that job immediately and it took me a while to find another job.

My mother was abusive to all the children but most with me. She also taught me a lot such as how to keep the house clean, organized, cooking, and sewing. She was a very hard worker.

The first time she broke my heart was when I won a playset from school. I was so excited to show my mom but instead, she began to hit me and I had no idea what I did wrong. My mom was so good for many things but at the same time also very abusive. When I was six I had a bathroom accident and my mom put me in a cold shower and began to beat me. I was not allowed to go to events with the family such as the circus, pool, bowling ally or family parties. I would have to help my siblings to get ready and I would be left at home. She would often beat me with me with a broom or belt. She told me I was no good bringing my self-esteem down. This impacted me later in life because I didn't feel like I deserved to have a good life.

I always enjoyed visiting my family but unfortunately, not everyone was nice. My male cousin tried to rape me twice. On one occasion after 15 min of physically fighting him, I was able to defend myself. Thankfully he did not hurt me. I told my female cousin (his sister) what happened and she defended me. She was shocked that her brother would try to do such a thing.

As a young adult, I experienced several incidents of violence. I was excited to go to the club one night, knowing that an architect I admired was going to be there. When he invited me to his apartment to review some design plans, I was thrilled. However, things took a dark turn when he began to smoke and tried to sexually assault me. Despite my protests, he continued, telling me that no one would believe me if I spoke out. In a moment of courage, I fought back, causing him to become even more agitated. I managed to escape the situation, but the emotional trauma lingered long after. When I was living in an apartment with friends, I faced another terrifying experience. One of the housemates attempted to sexually assault me, leading me to fight him off and find a hiding spot in a garage for hours. The fear and anxiety of being discovered weighed heavily on my mind as I sat in silence, waiting for the danger to pass. At one point, I worked at a school for children. One of my responsibilities was to complete the free lunch application. I had a very manipulative supervisor who demanded unethical behavior to increase funding for the school's free lunch program. I refused to comply with her demands and would often be yelled at. As a young woman in New York City, I would experience sexual violence on the trains. Three men exposed themselves to me. On one occasion I was able to tell a transit police officer and the man was arrested.

Reflecting on my past, I now have a deeper understanding of my father, mother, and all of the abusive encounters of my life. I've come to realize my father was also abused, which has helped me forgive him for the beatings and abandonment. Growing up, I was so focused on pleasing my parents that I neglected my well-being, a consequence of the abuse I endured. In adulthood, I sought out similar unhealthy relationships, hoping to find the love I was missing, when in reality I was just trying to fill an internal void. Despite the challenges I faced, I remained resilient and determined to stand up for myself and do what was right, even in the face of adversity.

Interviewer: When you were in the abuse, what were your coping mechanisms?

PR: As a kid I loved to listen to rock music. As an adult, I used to watch TV and talk with my mom on the phone.

Interviewer: What were your losses, (ie. Dreams, home, family…)?

PR: My art. My second abusive partner forced me to discard numerous art supplies, books, and my drawing table, leading me to shut down my business. Since entering that toxic relationship, I have not touched my airbrush, though I still possess it. Hopefully, I will one-day resume painting.

Interviewer: Who did you first reach out to, and what were their responses? Describe the professionals and personal people in your life that you reached out to.

PR: During my second abusive relationship, I first went to the police and reported the abuse. They advised me to get an order of protection, which I did. However, I then learned that I had to personally serve the order to my abusive partner. Fearing retaliation, I devised a plan to safely leave the situation. I first secured a storage unit and then called a moving company. When my partner left for the day, I knew I had limited time to move all my belongings before he returned. I was incredibly anxious, knowing that if my escape plan went wrong, he would likely hurt me severely.

The day before I escaped I went to the police precinct and they served him. Shaken, I went to a diner and broke down in tears. The movers ended up running late, but once they arrived, they worked quickly to pack up my things. I left my apartment key in the mailbox and then departed. My partner immediately began violating the order, texting and contacting me. I then went to the Family Justice Center and requested emergency shelter.

Interviewer: What were 3 defining moments that made you decide to seek help?

PR: There was no defining moment.

An immigration organization assisted me in accessing my first domestic violence shelter. During an interview, I disclosed that I was in an abusive relationship, a decision that ultimately led me to safety. After confiding in the organization about the abuse, they connected me with a social worker who helped me safely store my important belongings. In weekly counseling sessions, the social worker and I developed a plan for me to safely exit the abusive relationship—a plan that saved my life. The abuse escalated around this time. My husband raped me 3 times. When I asked for the divorce, he told me he would kill me first and then himself instead of signing the divorce papers. He was always yelling. One time, I asked him to clean a drinking glass and instead, he broke the glass and told me that's what I get. He would prevent me from leaving the house. He often threatened to kill me and burn down the building we were living in. The violence escalated to the point where my partner nearly killed me with a hammer. Fearing for my life, I recognized it was time to flee and I escaped to the first available shelter. Life in the shelter presented significant challenges—shared living spaces, lack of privacy, and limited staff support, despite their earnest efforts. Desperate to leave the shelter, I unwittingly entered into a new abusive relationship.

My second abuser, I believe was narcissistic. He would get very mad when I would say no to having sex. He would often force himself on me. At times I felt like I was just an object to have sex with. That's all that mattered to him. The first surgery I had was on my foot. He would not help at all. He would get mad at me when we were out in public and would say, "you will see when we get home." I paid for everything, cleaned, and cooked. He had no compassion. On one occasion he got mad at me and pushed me hard to the floor. I fell and hit my head on the table. When I told him he hurt me he said, "I didn't push you. You just fell. You know that." I felt very isolated. He did not permit me to bring anyone to the house or have any friends. He allowed my sister to visit the house three times but during the last visit he kicked her out and she did not come back again. When we would visit his parents I would only be able to speak when he was in the room with us.

I wasn't feeling well one day. I recall watching TV and feeling dizzy. I went to the bathroom, and several hours passed before I woke up. I called my mom, and she told me to eat something, so I made some soup. However, I still felt very sick, so I went to the hospital. I later learned that I had experienced a seizure and a brain tumor, requiring immediate surgery. I spent several weeks recovering in the hospital. While in the hospital, my partner visited me briefly on three occasions. During this time, I had ample opportunity to reflect on my next steps. On the day of my discharge, my partner picked me up and assured the doctor he would care for me at home. The doctors and nurses gave him clear instructions to help me with bathing, cooking, and daily tasks so I did not have to lift any heavy objects. My abuser took a paid 12-week Family Medical Leave (FMLA) from his job to "care for me." The surgeon agreed to this arrangement but the abuser never let anybody into the home to help me. However, once we arrived, he insisted I have sex with him and made me walk to the supermarket and carry the groceries back, despite the nurse's instructions for me to rest and avoid lifting heavy objects. I was in an incredible amount of pain. My abuser had a vacation for 3 months telling people he was helping me. He also yelled at me to take my medications. He always reminded me to tell people that he was taking good care of me and if I told the truth he would hurt me. Ultimately, I realized this was my second abusive relationship. I knew I deserved better and needed to regain control of my life. This experience left me feeling lost and broken, but I was determined to start over and create a healthier future for myself.

Interviewer: What were the barriers to reaching out for assistance/help?

PR: I was appalled when the police and court informed me that I was responsible for figuring out a way to serve the protective order on the individual who had been abusing me. I did not have anyone to severe the document so I went to the police and asked them to serve the document.

Despite the many hospital staff who could have intervened, no one asked me about the abuse I was suffering, and I was too afraid to speak up. Afterward, I often wondered what they thought about the lack of visits from my abuser. I wish the hospital had insisted on arranging home health care or regular check-ins to ensure my well-being.

Interviewer: How did the abuse affect your physical and mental health?

PR: After seeking refuge in a second shelter, I was overcome by a deep sense of depression and anxiety. The emotional turmoil manifested physically, as I began experiencing regular seizures that required frequent hospital visits and doctor consultations to manage my deteriorating health. I recognized that my mental well-being was the root cause of these physical problems.

It was during my extended stay at the shelter that I was eventually connected with supportive housing. The transition to my new home was daunting; I was gripped by fear and would often simply lie in bed, crying. I was experiencing intense panic attacks and severe anxiety. I slept the day away. At my lowest point, I was taking an astonishing 32 medications per day.

One pivotal day, I decided to adopt a dog. This decision proved transformative—caring for my new companion compelled me to get up, go for walks, and attend to his needs. The joy and companionship he provided were instrumental in my gradual recovery. There are still days when I struggle to leave my bed, but the responsibility of caring for my dog motivates me to push forward.

I have also discovered the therapeutic benefits of gardening. On the rooftop of my supportive housing, I have cultivated an abundance of produce, including tomatoes, potatoes, corn, peppers, basil, and parsley. Sharing these homegrown bounties with my community has been a source of immense fulfillment.

Today, I am proud to say that I am completely free of medication and feel a profound sense of peace and vitality. My journey has been arduous, but the decision to welcome a furry friend and embrace the restorative power of nature has helped me reclaim my life.

Interviewer: What systems did you engage with through your process of healing, (ie. Medical, psychiatric/**psychological, social work, shelter, financial, housing, legal, spiritual, etc.)**

PR: Over the years, many people have helped me through difficult times.

The social workers, psychiatrist, and nurse at the second shelter were incredibly supportive—they listened to me and ensured I received the medical care I desperately needed. The case managers then helped me find my own home. At the supportive housing program, the staff always makes time to listen and help me with tasks like gardening. I also feel a sense of safety knowing the front desk staff is there to monitor who comes and goes. Additionally, an amazing psychiatrist helped me understand the connection between my medical conditions and my depression/anxiety. The psychiatrist made me feel stronger. He would listen to me and let me cry freely.

Interviewer: What were the top two systems that aided in your healing?

PR: The shelter and supportive housing.

Interviewer: Looking back at your experience and everything you went through, what advice would you give to others to help in their healing? (Her pearls for others).

PR:

- Don't be afraid to ask for help. Trust yourself, believe in yourself, be your own best friend, and never stop dreaming about what you want to do and your goals.

- Don't think that people who are abused didn't go to school. Anyone can be abused. It doesn't matter your skin color, gender, education, etc. ANYONE
- If you think you can, then you will. If you think you cannot, then you won't.
- Healing is a complex process. It is many things together.
- Forgiveness is very important because that way you can get peace and harmony in your life.
- Loving yourself is the first step to taking better care of yourself. Without self-love, it's all too easy to repeat the same mistakes. This journey is not simple and will require time and effort. However, if you are truly committed, you will learn how to love and care for yourself. Love yourself before anyone else. When we love ourselves first, we are not looking for love somewhere else.
- Conduct thorough research to learn about the resources available to help you move on and escape from an abusive relationship. Explore online sources, speak with counselors at your child's school, consult your doctor or a social worker at the hospital, and utilize any other relevant avenues of information.
- It's important to speak up, but be selective about whom you confide in. Avoid sharing details with the family members or friends of your abuser, as this may not be a safe or productive conversation.
- Enjoy being by yourself. Know yourself—what you can and cannot do. Accept who you are, good and bad. Surround yourself with people who will bring you joy.
- "What you think of me is not my business."
  - When a person starts healing there will always be people who do not like to see you happy.

Interviewer: How are you doing today?

PR: I am grateful to have found a sense of peace. Every day I choose to live in the present I have forgiven every one that has hurt me. I am glad to share my story in the hopes of helping others who have endured similar experiences.

Survivors are whole individuals with complex and complicated histories and coping skills. Sometimes when we see individuals in their older years, we often see their frailty, limited mobility, diminished ability to express themselves verbally, and their isolated state. Older Adults are a culmination of their entire life. Understanding how someone came to be who they are as your patient or client is very important. Meeting the older adult where they are and adhering to and respecting their wishes, acknowledges them as whole human beings and allows you as the professional to engage with them humanely and respectfully. Obtaining important information about the survivor's abuse and history can help save someone's life.

A special thanks to all survivors. Your strength, resilience, and knowledge cannot be overstated or overlooked.

Correction to: Elder Abuse and Neglect

Veronica LoFaso and Lisa Rachmuth

Correction to:
V. LoFaso, L. Rachmuth (eds.), *Elder Abuse and Neglect*, https://doi.org/10.1007/978-3-031-97784-8

The book was inadvertently published with an incorrect author name as "Susan Shulman Roth" in the acknowledgements section. Now, it has been updated as "Susan Shulman" in the book.

The updated version of this book can be found at
https://doi.org/10.1007/978-3-031-97784-8

V. LoFaso, L. Rachmuth (eds.), *Elder Abuse and Neglect*,
https://doi.org/10.1007/978-3-031-97784-8_12

Index

V. LoFaso, L. Rachmuth (eds.), *Elder Abuse and Neglect*,
https://doi.org/10.1007/978-3-031-97784-8

G

H

S

T

U

MIX
Papier aus verantwortungsvollen Quellen
Paper from responsible sources
FSC® C105338

If you have any concerns about our products,
you can contact us on
ProductSafety@springernature.com

In case Publisher is established outside the EU,
the EU authorized representative is:
Springer Nature Customer Service Center GmbH
Europaplatz 3, 69115 Heidelberg, Germany

Printed by Libri Plureos GmbH
in Hamburg, Germany